Fundamentals of Optometry

Refraction, Dispensing Optics and Ophthalmic Procedures

Fundamentals of Optometry

Refraction, Dispensing Optics and Ophthalmic Procedures

Second Edition

Ashwani Kumar Ghai MS
Senior Consultant (Eye Surgeon)
NKS Super Speciality Hospital
Gulabi Bagh, New Delhi, India
Mojiram Lions Eye Hospital
Akbarpur Majra, Delhi, India
Dr Ashwani Ghai Eye Care Clinic
Rohini, New Delhi, India

Forewords
Rajender Singh Chauhan
Rajesh Sinha

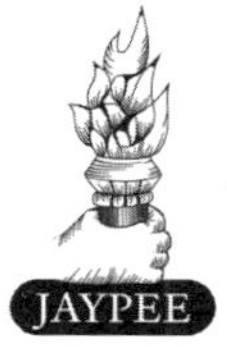

JAYPEE BROTHERS MEDICAL PUBLISHERS
The Health Sciences Publisher
New Delhi | London

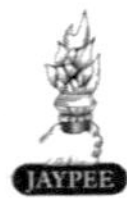

Jaypee Brothers Medical Publishers (P) Ltd

Headquarters
Jaypee Brothers Medical Publishers (P) Ltd
EMCA House, 23/23-B
Ansari Road, Daryaganj
New Delhi 110 002, India
Landline: +91-11-23272143, +91-11-23272703
+91-11-23282021, +91-11-23245672
Email: jaypee@jaypeebrothers.com

Corporate Office
Jaypee Brothers Medical Publishers (P) Ltd
4838/24, Ansari Road, Daryaganj
New Delhi 110 002, India
Phone: +91-11-43574357
Fax: +91-11-43574314
Email: jaypee@jaypeebrothers.com

Overseas Office
J.P. Medical Ltd
83 Victoria Street, London
SW1H 0HW (UK)
Phone: +44 20 3170 8910
Fax: +44 (0)20 3008 6180
Email: info@jpmedpub.com

Website: www.jaypeebrothers.com
Website: www.jaypeedigital.com

Inquiries for bulk sales may be solicited at: jaypee@jaypeebrothers.com

Fundamentals of Optometry: Refraction, Dispensing Optics and Ophthalmic Procedures

First Edition: 2013

Second Edition: **2025**

ISBN: 978-93-5696-827-1

Printed in India at Sterling Graphics Pvt. Ltd.

Dedicated to

My *late* parents for their blessings
and
My wife Dr Reena Ghai and my son Ayush Ghai
for their patience and understanding

Contributors

Manisha Nada
Professor
Department of Ophthalmology
Regional Institute of Ophthalmology
Post Graduate Institute of Medical Sciences
Rohtak, Haryana, India
(Chapter 13: Lasers in Ophthalmology)

Nikita Sethi
Assistant Professor
Master of Optometry (Amity University)
SGT University
Gurugram, Haryana, India
(Chapter 9: Ophthalmic Lenses and Chapter 14: Contact Lens Practice)

Foreword

Optometry is more than just diagnosing refractive errors; it is about understanding the intricate interaction of ocular health, visual perception, and quality of life. As practitioners, optometrists are at the forefront of vision care, entrusted with the critical task of preserving and enhancing one of our most precious senses, the sense of sight.

This book serves as an invaluable resource for both aspiring and practicing optometrists alike. From the foundational principles of properties of light and refractive errors to advanced diagnostic techniques and emerging technologies, each chapter is meticulously crafted to provide a deep dive into the multifaceted world of optometric practice.

I commend the author for his dedication to advancing the field of optometry and for creating a resource that will undoubtedly inspire the next generation of eye care professionals. May this book serve as a guiding light, empowering you to deliver compassionate, evidence-based care that transforms the lives of your patients. I have no doubt that this book will elicit a lot of appreciation and acceptance by both optometrists and residents. This will be a real tribute to the hard work the author has put into writing the book.

Prepare to embark on a transformative learning experience—one that celebrates the art and science of optometry in all its dimensions. Your commitment to excellence in vision care starts here.

Rajender Singh Chauhan
MBBS MS
Senior Professor and Head
Department of Ophthalmology
Regional Institute of Ophthalmology
Post Graduate Institute of Medical Sciences
Rohtak, Haryana, India

Foreword

Welcome to the world of optometry, where the science of vision meets the art of care. In *Fundamentals of Optometry: Refraction, Dispensing Optics and Ophthalmic Procedures*, we embark on a journey through the essential principles and practices that underpin this critical field of healthcare.

Vision is not merely the ability to see but a complex interplay of biological processes, optics, and neurological pathways. Understanding these intricacies forms the cornerstone of effective optometric practice. This book is meticulously crafted to equip both students and practitioners with a comprehensive framework—from the basic knowledge of properties of light to advanced diagnostic techniques like OCT and pentacam—that ensures every patient receives the highest standard of care.

Optometry is a profession that blends technical expertise with compassion. It requires not only a deep understanding of ocular health and vision correction but also a dedication to improving the quality of life for each individual who seeks our help. As such, this book not only delves into the scientific fundamentals but also emphasizes the human dimension of optometric practice, reminding us that behind every diagnosis and prescription lies a person deserving our empathy and respect.

In these pages, you will find a synthesis of current research, clinical insights, and practical wisdom accumulated from decades of collective experience. It is our hope that *Fundamentals of Optometry: Refraction, Dispensing Optics and Ophthalmic Procedures*, serves as a trusted guide, inspiring both new and seasoned professionals to uphold the highest standards of patient care and to continually advance the frontiers of knowledge in our field.

As you embark on your journey through this book, may you discover the profound impact that optometry can have on individuals and communities alike. May it ignite your curiosity, deepen your understanding, and reaffirm your commitment to the noble pursuit of preserving and enhancing vision for all.

Rajesh Sinha
MD DNB FIACLE FRCS
Professor
Department of Cornea
Lens and Refractive Surgery Services
RP Centre, AIIMS, New Delhi, India

Preface to the Second Edition

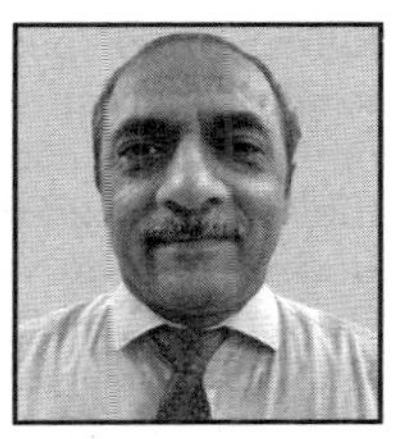

It is with great pleasure and enthusiasm that I present the second edition of *Fundamentals of Optometry: Refraction, Dispensing Optics and Ophthalmic Procedures.* Since the publication of the first edition, the field of optometry has been revolutionized a lot, driven by advancements in technology, changes in healthcare delivery, and a deeper understanding of ocular conditions and their management.

This edition builds upon the strong foundation laid down in the first edition, aiming to provide optometry students, practitioners, and allied healthcare professionals with a comprehensive and up-to-date knowledge of the subject.

Key updates in this edition include:

- **Expanded coverage:** Expanded content on emerging topics such as myopia management, and advancements in contact lens technology.
- **Technological advances:** Integration of the latest diagnostic tools and therapeutic approaches as per needs of the industry.

As in the first edition, our goal remains to foster a deep understanding of the fundamental concepts while preparing the reader to navigate the complexities of modern optometric practice. This book continues to serve as both a foundational text for students and a practical reference for seasoned professionals.

I am deeply grateful to my colleagues, students, and mentors whose invaluable insights and feedback have shaped this edition. Their commitment to advancing the field of optometry has been instrumental in ensuring the relevance and accuracy of the content.

Finally, I hope that this book inspires readers to explore, innovate, and uphold the highest standards of patient care. Whether you are beginning your journey in optometry or seeking to deepen your expertise, I trust that *Fundamentals of Optometry: Refraction, Dispensing Optics and Ophthalmic Procedures, Second Edition* will serve as a trusted companion in your pursuit of excellence.

Ashwani Kumar Ghai

Preface to the First Edition

Refraction, Dispensing Optics and Ophthalmic Procedures is a book written to take care of students of optometry, ophthalmic technicians and practicing opticians. The contents of the book have been designed taking into account the syllabus laid down by All India Institute of Medical Sciences (AIIMS), Indira Gandhi National Open University (IGNOU), Vinayaka Missions University (VMU), Allahabad Agricultural Institute, and Institute of Public Health and Hygiene (IPH&H), and other prestigious institutes, for students of optometry. However, it will be of equal use to students of MBBS course and ophthalmology residents.

The book has been written in a very simple language and to the point. Many illustrations have been given to explain the matter in a better way, wherever, required. All efforts have been made to explain the significance of the phenomenon in our day-to-day life, wherever relevant.

I have made all possible efforts to check the correctness of the text material. Still, I feel such ventures are not likely to be free from human errors, certain inaccuracies, etc., for which, I apologize sincerely. Therefore, feedbacks from all those who go through the material will help improve future editions. An endeavor of this kind will be highly appreciated and duly acknowledged.

Ashwani Kumar Ghai

Acknowledgments

First of all, I would like to express my gratitude to Professor (Dr) Md Ejaz Hussain, Dean, Faculty of Allied Health Sciences, for his constant encouragement and guidance that helped me achieve this goal.

I would like to thank the policy makers of SGT University who promote every single instance of innovation and publications under able guidance and leadership of Mrs Madhu Preet Kaur Chawla, Chairperson, and Mr Man Mohan Singh Chawla, Managing Trustee.

I would like to thank my senior colleagues Dr Neeraj Sharma, Professor and Head, Department of Ophthalmology, SGT University, Gurugram, Haryana; Dr JP Chugh, Senior Professor, Department of Ophthalmology and my mentor, SGT University, Gurugram; Dr Vibha Jha, Head, Department of Paramedical Sciences and all other staff members of the university for providing me the favorable environment.

My sincere thanks to Dr Neha Mohan, Retina Specialist, Jain Eye Hospital and Laser Centre, Shalimar Bagh, New Delhi, and Dr Rakesh Mahajan, Comprehensive Ophthalmologist, Mahajan Eye Centre, Pitampura, New Delhi, for providing me with good-quality images for academic purposes.

I am also indebted to my publishers M/s Jaypee Brothers Medical Publishers (P) Ltd, New Delhi, India, who helped and guided me, Shri Jitendar P Vij (Group Chairman), Mr Ankit Vij (Managing Director), Mr MS Mani (Group President), Dr Madhu Choudhary (Director—Educational Publishing), Ms Pooja Bhandari [Director—Production (Books and Journals)], Ms Sunita Katla (Executive Assistant to Group Chairman and Publishing Manager), Ms Samina Khan (Executive Assistant to Director—Educational Publishing), Dr Upma Tomar (Senior Development Editor), Mr Ajay Kumar Sharma [DGM (Books and Journals)], Ms Seema Dogra (Cover Visualizer), Ms Neha Verma (Graphic Designer—Cover), Mr Rajesh Sharma (Production Coordinator), Ms Geeta Barik (Proofreader), Mr Mahesh Chand Joshi (Typesetter), and Mr Nitesh Jain (Graphic Designer), for all their support to work in this project and make it a success. Without their cooperation, I could not have completed this project.

I would like to thank my students who have been a constant source of encouragement that turned this dream into reality.

Contents

PLATE 1

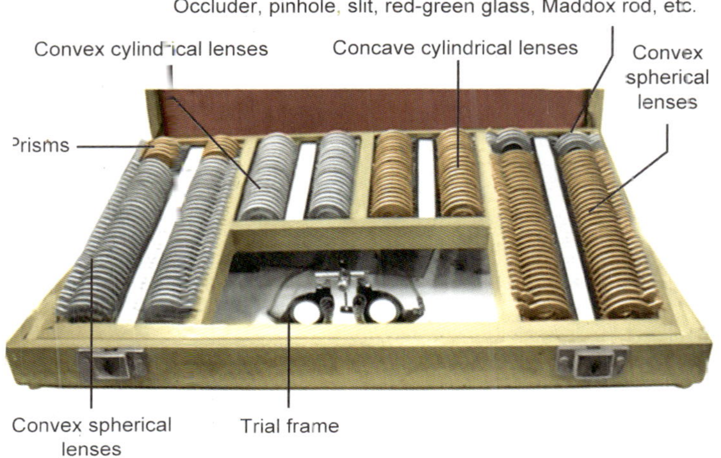

Fig. 3.1: Trial set

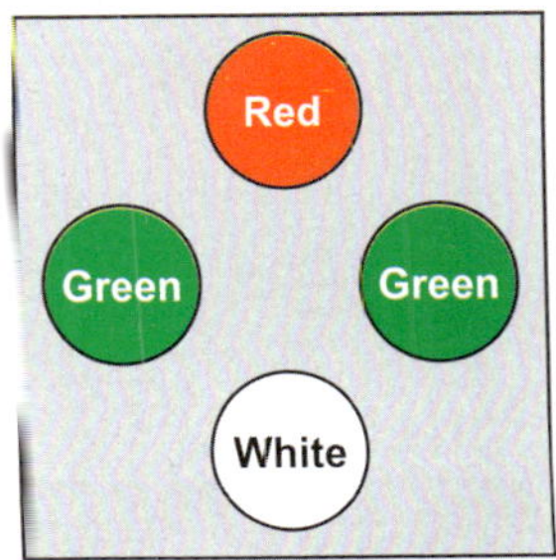

Fig. 3.5: Worth's four dot test

PLATE 2

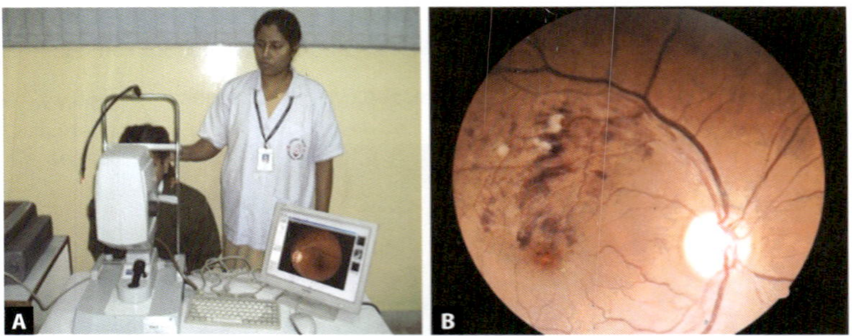

Figs. 12.8A and B: (A) Fundus camera; (B) Fundus photograph.

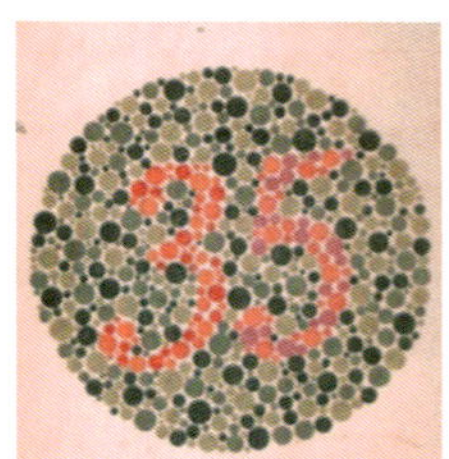

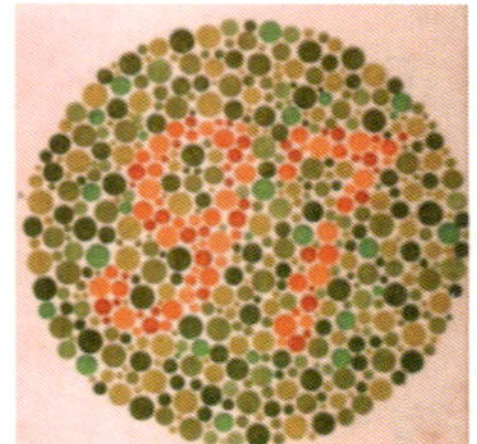

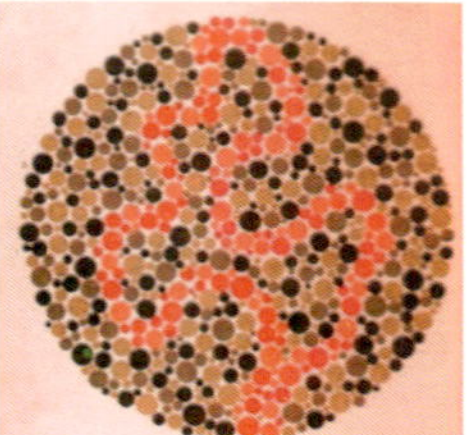

Fig. 12.35: Ishihara charts

1 CHAPTER

Light

WHAT IS LIGHT?

Light is a form of energy to which human eye is sensitive. The whole electromagnetic spectrum ranges from cosmic rays on shorter wavelength to radio waves on longer wavelength **(Fig. 1.1)**. Ultraviolet rays, infrared rays and visible rays are clinically significant from an ophthalmic point of view. Visible white light consists of seven colors ranging from violet (400 nanometer) to red (700 nanometer). Light with longer wavelength has lesser energy and light with shorter wavelength has more energy.

Optics is a branch of physics which deals with properties of light including its interaction with matter and construction of instruments that use or detect it.

ULTRAVIOLET RAYS

Ultraviolet (UV) rays are invisible rays, sunlight being the principal source. Depending upon their absorption spectrum, UV light has been divided into three bands:

1. **Ultraviolet A rays:** This band of UV rays is absorbed by crystalline lens and thus retina is protected against their bad effects. Prolonged exposure to these rays causes cataract formation. IOLs implanted during cataract surgery have chromophores (inhibitors of UV rays) to protect retina against UV rays.
2. **Ultraviolet B rays:** This band is responsible for snow blindness and photokeratitis caused by welding arc. Prolonged exposure to these rays can cause formation of pinguecula and pterygium.
3. **Ultraviolet C rays:** This band is blocked by the ozone layer of atmosphere.

Cosmic rays	Gamma rays	X-ray	Ultraviolet rays	Visible rays	Infrared rays	Micro waves	Radar waves	Radio waves
10^{-6} nm	10^{-3} nm	.01- 10 nm	C B A	VIBGYOR	C B A	10^4	10^6	10^9
200 nm → Optical Radiations ← 10^4 nm								

Fig. 1.1: Electromagnetic spectrum of light.

VISIBLE RAYS

It consists of violet, indigo, blue, green, yellow, orange, and red light. Red color has longest wavelength. That is why traffic signals are made of red light so that it is visible from a long distance. Retina is most sensitive to yellow light in photopic conditions. In scotopic conditions it is most sensitive to blue light.

INFRARED RAYS

These rays are absorbed in anterior chamber and cause heating effect. They are also called as heat rays. They are further of three types:

- Infrared A rays are responsible for macular burn in solar eclipse (photo retinitis).
- Infrared rays B and C can cause corneal opacity and cataract formation on prolonged exposure.

PROPAGATION OF LIGHT

Light travels in all directions in straight lines from the source of light. It travels in the form of waves that oscillate in all directions and also in form of tiny particles called photons. A *photon* is an elementary particle and the basic unit of light and all other forms of electromagnetic radiation. It has no rest mass. It shows dual nature, i.e., it exhibits properties of both waves and particles. For example, a single photon is refracted by a lens and exhibits wave interference with itself. The modern concept of the photon was developed by Einstein to explain experimental observations that did not fit the classical wave model of light **(Fig. 1.2)**.

Thus light has dual nature. The term "ray" is used for the path along which the light travels. It is represented by a straight line. A bundle of rays is called a pencil or a beam of light.

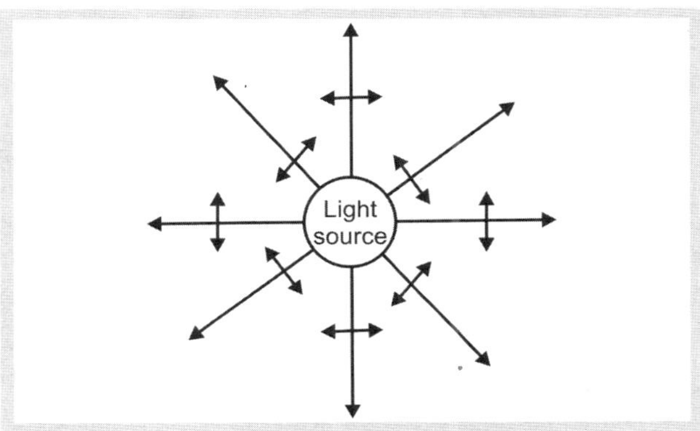

Fig. 1.2: Propagation of light.

Rays of light may have *positive vergence,* i.e., when they travel, they converge at a point or *negative vergence,* i.e., when they travel, they diverge from a point or they may have *zero vergence,* i.e., they are running parallel to each other **(Fig. 1.3)**.

A medium through which light can pass uninterrupted is called *transparent medium*. A medium which offers some resistance to the passage of light is called *translucent medium* and a medium which does not allow passage of light through it is called the *opaque medium*.

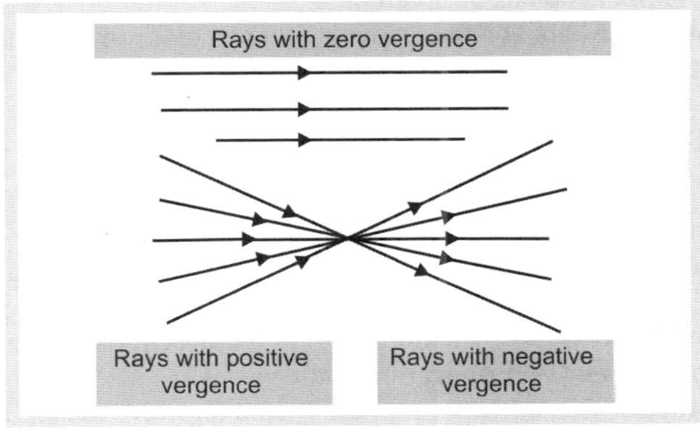

Fig. 1.3: Vergence of rays.

SPEED OF LIGHT

Speed of light is the fastest anything has been observed to move. In vacuum, the speed is three lakh kilometers per second or one lakh eighty six thousand miles per second. At this speed, it takes light one ten thousandth of a second to travel around the earth. When light enters a material, it slows down. The amount depends on the material it enters and its density. For example, light travels about 30% slower in water than it does in a vacuum, while in diamonds, which is about the densest material, it travels at about half the speed it does in a vacuum.

HOW DO WE SEE?

Sun is the natural source of light. When light falls on a nonluminous body, following things can happen:

- Light strikes the surface, some part of it is absorbed and some part is reflected back. This reflected part of light enters our eyeball and stimulates our rods and cones which generate a visual impulse. This is carried via optic nerve to visual cortex where the signals are interpreted. Image formed on retina is very small and inverted which is reinverted and made of original size in the visual cortex. A red object appears red because it absorbs colors of all wavelengths and reflects red color which enters our eye to generate a sensation of red color.
- Whole of the light is absorbed and no color is reflected back, the object appears black or opaque.
- Whole of the light is reflected back and no color are absorbed, the object appears white.

HUYGENS' PRINCIPLE

The Dutch physicist Christiaan Huygens and French physicist Augustin Jean Fresnel were the two scientists who gave this principle. It is used to analyze problems of wave propagation. According to this principle every point of a wave front may be considered as the source of secondary wavelets that spread out in all directions with a speed equal to the speed of propagation of the waves.

This means that each point of an advancing wave acts as a fresh source of waves creating a series of circular wave. Thus, as the wave advances, each advancing wave in turn creates next stream of successive waves and so on. It can be thought of as an example given below:

If two rooms are connected through an open door and you create a sound in the extreme corner of one room (farthest from the other room), to any person sitting in the second room, it will appear as if the sound has been created from the door (or starting point of the second room) itself. It is because when a person creates a sound in one room, the wave travels ahead and the next wave again creates the stream of waves. This continues and passes the person sitting in the second room. The person assumes as if the sound is created from the entry of the door itself.

Applications

- Diffraction refers to various phenomena which occur when a wave encounters an obstacle. It is described as the apparent bending of waves around small obstacles and the spreading out of waves past small openings. Now, this can be explained through Huygens' principle. When the wave hits an obstacle, the points where it touches the obstacle through the slit, start creating waves in all directions. Waves moving in the same direction are added together. Hence, it appears as if waves are spreading out of small opening.
- *Reflection and refraction:* When a ray (or wave) hits a surface, the point at which it hits, starts creating waves. If the upper medium has different refractive index than the lower medium, we see the size in the waves as different. The tangent of these waves explains the angle of reflection and refraction.

PROPERTIES OF LIGHT

Until the middle of 1800s, light was taken to be a stream of tiny particles. This was advocated by Newton. However, by the late 1800s, the particle theory was replaced by the wave theory. This was because light exhibited certain properties that could only be explained by the wave theory. Now the most accepted view is that light exhibits dual nature. Different properties of light are:

- Reflection
- Refraction
- Total internal reflection

- Dispersion
- Diffraction
- Polarization
- Interference

Reflection

When a ray of light strikes a polished surface, it bounces back in a particular direction. This is known as reflection of light. Light ray falling on the surface is called *incident ray*, the ray that bounces back is called the *reflected ray* and a line drawn at right angle to the surface is called *normal* **(Fig. 1.4)**. This phenomenon allows us to see images in mirrors. We see the images in mirrors as apparently coming from behind the mirror because our eyes interpret it in this manner. But when we see ourselves reflected in the mirror and raise our left arm, the image apparently raises its right arm. This is because the image is laterally reversed.

Laws of Reflection

The laws of reflection can be summarized as:

- The incident ray, the reflected ray and the normal at the point of incidence, all lie in the same plane.
- The angle of incidence is equal to the angle of reflection.

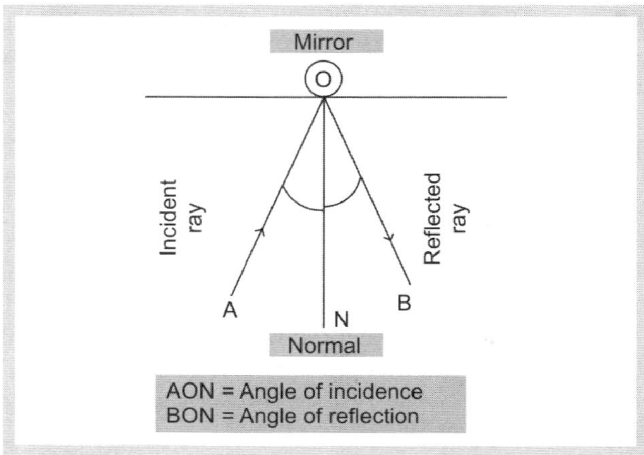

Fig. 1.4: Reflection of light.

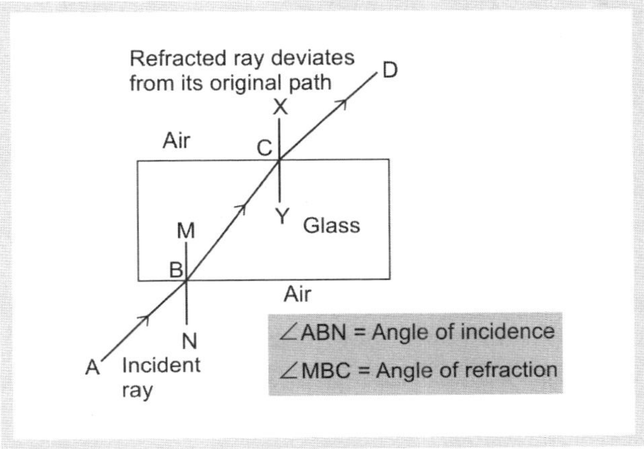

Fig. 1.5: Refraction of light.

Refraction

When a ray of light passes from one medium (say air) to another medium (say glass) of different optical density, it deviates from its original path. This is called refraction. When it passes from denser to rarer medium it deviates away from normal and when it passes from rarer medium to denser medium it deviates towards normal. The greater the density difference between the two media, the more the light bends. This property is used in optical lenses used to correct refractive errors and to make different ophthalmic instruments **(Fig. 1.5)**.

Refraction Through a Plate of Glass

When a ray of light passes through a denser medium its speed is slowed down. It does not deviate from its path if it strikes the denser medium at right angle to it. But if it strikes the medium obliquely, it deviates from its path as shown in **Figures 1.6 and 1.7**.

When we look into the surface of a lake or pond while fishing, the fish we catch seems larger when under the water than when we actually land it. This is due to refraction. Since the air is less dense than water, the light bends away from the normal as it emerges out of water to enter our eyes. This is the reason that stars twinkle and if a wooden stick is half dipped in water, the underwater portion of stick appears broken.

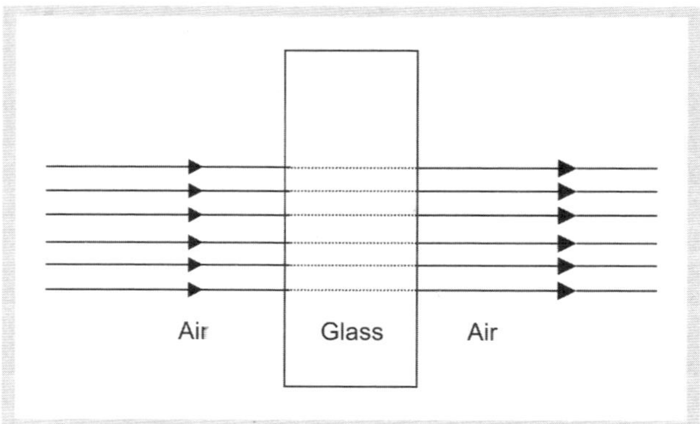

Fig. 1.6: Refraction through plate of glass.

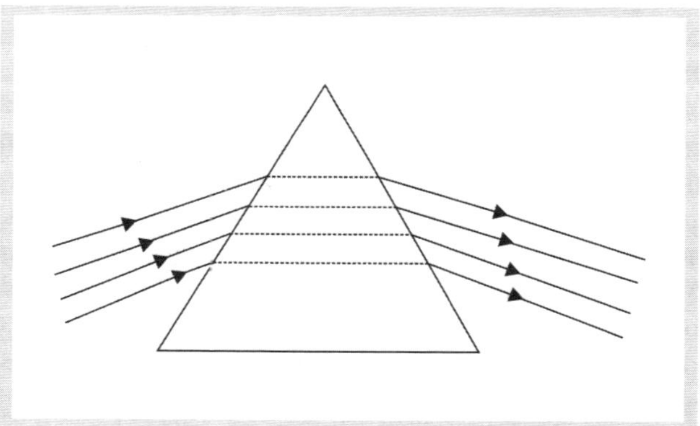

Fig. 1.7: Refraction through prism.

Laws of Refraction

- The incident ray and the refracted ray are on the opposite sides of the normal at the point of incidence and all three lie in the same plane.
- The ratio of sine of angle of incidence to the sine of angle of refraction is constant. This is known as *Snell's Law*. The value of this constant is known as refractive index of the medium. The refractive index of water is 1.33, crown glass is 1.52, flint glass is 1.65 and air is 1.00.

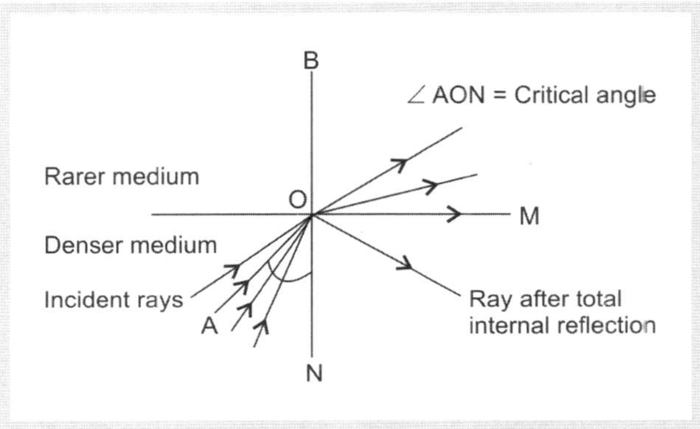

Fig. 1.8: Total internal reflection.

Total Internal Reflection

Another property that combines both refraction and reflection is *total internal reflection*. If for an incident ray of light angle of incidence is increased, its angle of refraction also increases. A limit comes when the refracted ray travels parallel to the surface. This angle of incidence for which angle of refraction is 90° is known as *critical angle*. If angle of incidence is increased further, the refracted ray bends and travels in the same medium. This is known as total internal reflection **(Fig. 1.8)**. This phenomenon is made use of in making optical fibers. Diamond shines even in dark because of this phenomenon. Fiber optics uses this property of light to keep light beams focused without significant loss, as long as the bending of the cable is not too sharp. TV and telephone cables use fiber optic cable more and more since it is much faster and more efficient than electrons in an electric current.

Dispersion or Polychromatic Effects of Light

It refers to the ability to break white light into its constituent colors. White light consists of seven colors. If white light enters a prism it splits into seven colors with violet light having shortest wavelength suffers maximum deviation and red light with longest wavelength suffers minimum deviation **(Fig. 1.9)**.

Rainbows are natural phenomena that exemplify all of the above properties of light. They use refraction, dispersion, and internal reflection to produce their amazing hues. White light enters

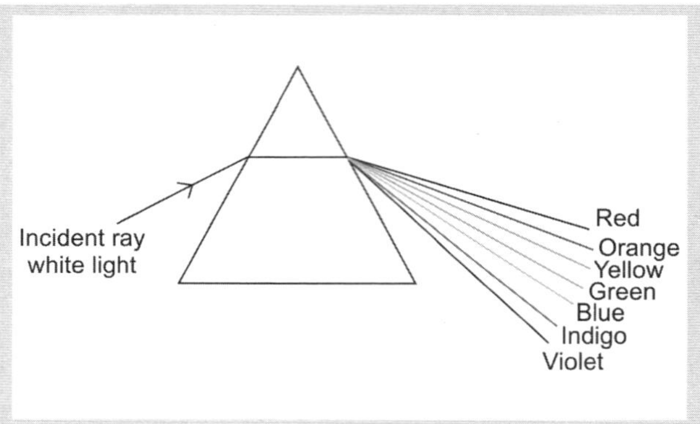

Fig. 1.9: Dispersion of light.

raindrops from the sun it gets dispersed and refracted inside the raindrops. When the dispersed light hits the back of the raindrop, it gets internally reflected, and when it emerges it gets dispersed even more.

The color you see most vividly in a rainbow depends on the angle of your eye. Generally, you must look higher in the sky to see the red, and lower to see the blue. What you actually see is the red on the top and the blue on the bottom, with all of the other colors in between. The arc of the rainbow depends on the angle that your line of sight makes relative to the sun behind you.

Diffraction

Diffraction refers to the fact that light bends as it goes through an opening. It is difficult to give an everyday example of this; an easier example is with another wave form, sound. When someone speaks from in front of an open door, a person standing way around the corner from the door will still hear the diffracted sound waves. The phenomenon of diffraction is more if the size of aperture is small and vice versa. This is the reason that diffraction is less if the pupil is dilated and it is more when the pupil is constricted.

Polarization

Polarization is another property of light. Since a light wave's electric field vibrates in a direction perpendicular to its propagation motion,

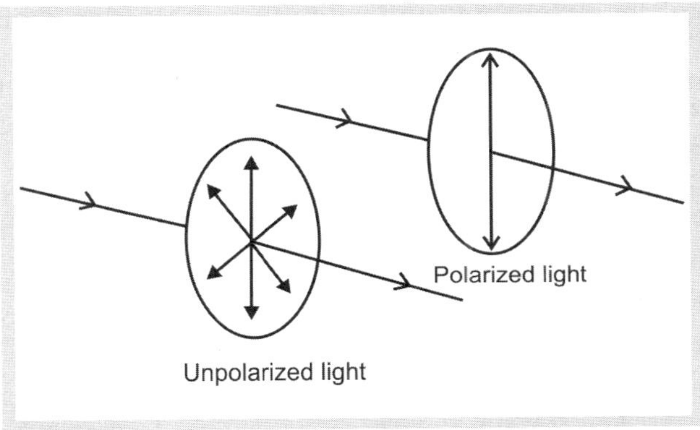

Fig. 1.10: Polarization of light.

it is called a transverse wave and is polarizable. A sound wave, by contrast, vibrates back and forth along its propagation direction and thus is not polarizable. Light is unpolarized if it is composed of vibrations in many different directions, with no preferred orientation. Many light sources (e.g., incandescent bulbs, arc lamps, and the sun) produce unpolarized light **(Fig. 1.10)**.

A common example of the use of polarization in our daily life is found in polarizing sunglasses. The material in the lenses passes light whose electric field vibrations are perpendicular to certain molecular alignments and absorbs light whose electric field vibrations are parallel to the molecular alignments. The major component of light reflecting from a surface, such as a lake or car hood, is horizontally polarized, parallel to the surface. Thus, polarization in sunglasses, with the transmission axis in a vertical direction, rejects horizontally polarized light and therefore reduces glare. However, if you consider a sunbather lying on his or her side, wearing such sunglasses, the usual vertical polarization (transmission axis) will now be at 90° and parallel to the surface and will therefore pass the horizontally polarized light reflected off the water or the land.

Interference

Interference is another property of light. It is a phenomenon that occurs when two beams of light meet. Depending on both the nature of the two beams and when they meet, they can either merge and enhance one another and give a brighter beam, or they might interfere in such a way as to make the merged beam less bright. The former is called constructive interference, and the latter is destructive interference **(Figs. 1.11 to 1.13)**. One experiment used to demonstrate how light signals can interfere with one another is called *Young's double slit experiment* after the physicist who used it for demonstrating the interference phenomenon **(Fig. 1.14)**.

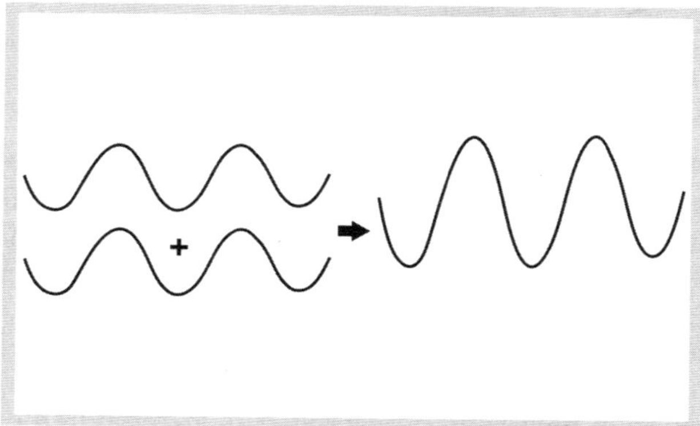

Fig. 1.11: Constructive interference.

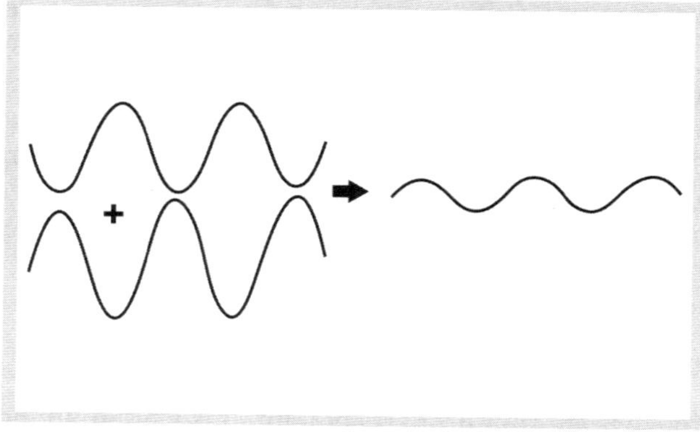

Fig. 1.12: Destructive interference.

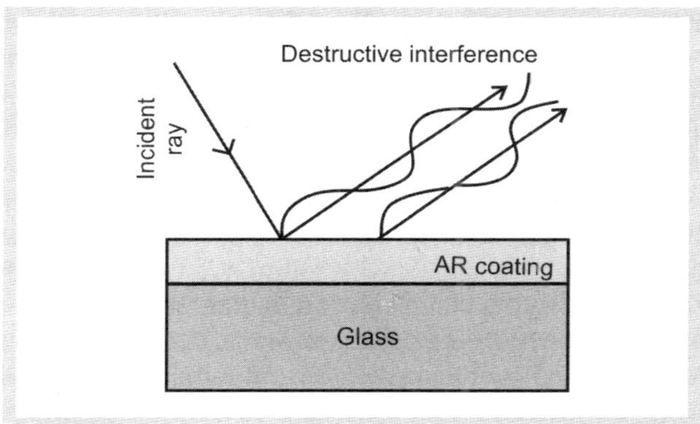

Fig. 1.13: Destructive interference in AR coating.

He set up a screen with two small slits and behind it set up another screen some distance away. When he subjected the first screen to a single light source, he found that there were alternate light and dark spots on the distance screen, corresponding to points where light rays coming from the two different slits underwent constructive and destructive interference. This is only possible when we think of light in terms of waves.

One situation that is illustrative of interference is where there is oil or gasoline floating on the surface of a puddle. Sometimes, you will

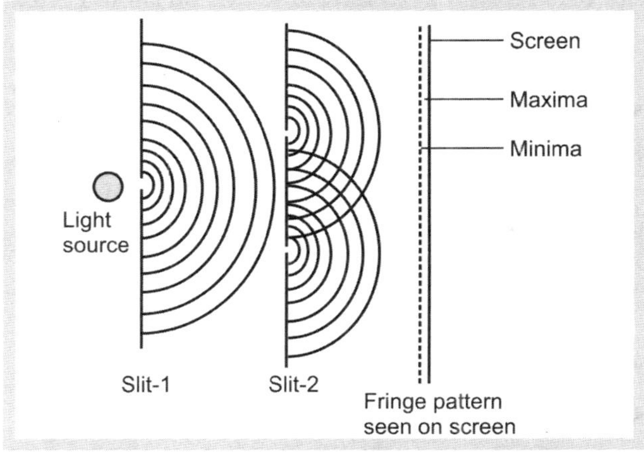

Fig. 1.14: Young's double slit experiment.

see a brilliant pattern of colors given off by the oil or gas, even when the gas or oil is subjected to white light. What happens is that different potions of the film cause different colors in the white light to interfere constructively or destructively, depending on the thickness of the film. One region of the film might look red because the red light bouncing off the top of the film interferes constructively with red light passing through the film and is then reflected back off the water below it.

We can see this more clearly with sound. When you are in the back of an auditorium, sound can reach you in different ways. It can take a direct path, be reflected off a ceiling, or walls, or the floor. All of these will reach you at slightly different times, and sometimes not at all. They can actually cancel each other out and you hear nothing when you sit in one area (also called dead zone), and sitting in another, you can hear an abnormally loud sound. These are examples of destructive and constructive interference and the reason that modern auditoriums use sound absorbing materials on ceilings, walls, and floors.

LASER INTERFEROMETER

Laser interferometer is an equipment meant clinically **(Fig. 1.15)** to determine outcome of a cataract surgery especially where cataract is mature or hyper mature. In this type of cataract, retinal details cannot be seen hence in spite of best surgery, outcome may not be rewarding due to associated macular pathology. Laser interferometry done prior to surgery, tells us how much vision should be expected.

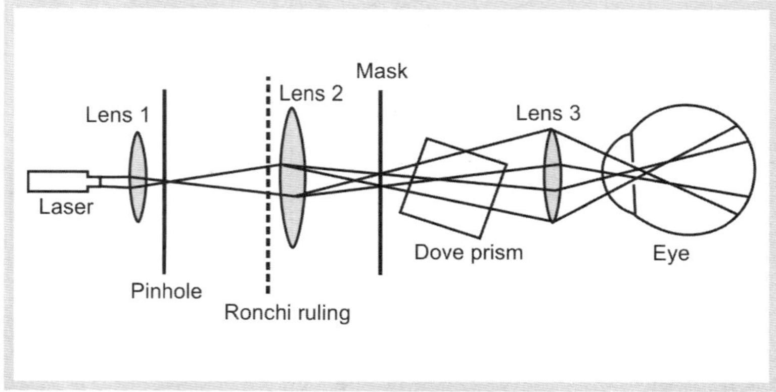

Fig. 1.15: Laser interferometer.

It is based on the principle of interference. Patient sees stripes whose size can be varied as desired. Depending upon size of stripe appreciated patient's vision can be assessed. However this test is more of academic importance and has not been able to gain any clinical significance because of its limitations.

LAW OF INVERSE SQUARE

This law applies to light, sound, electricity, gravitation, etc. It states that the intensity of light, i.e., luminance radiating from a point source is inversely proportional to the square of the distance from the source. So an object twice as far away receives only one quarter the energy in the same time period. In other words, we can say that the intensity of a spherical wavefront varies inversely with the square of the distance from the source assuming that there is no loss caused by absorption or scattering. For example, the intensity of radiation from Sun is 9140 watts per square meter at the distance of Mercury (0.387AU) but only 1370 watts per square meter at the distance of the Earth (1AU), i.e., a threefold increase in distance results in a nine fold decrease in intensity of radiation. For a point source, the equation is

$E = 1/d^2$; where E = Energy at one particular point
d = Distance of point from the source of light

Clinical Application

This law is made use of by photographers and theatrical professionals to determine optimum location of the light source for proper illumination of the subject. This law can be used only in case of a point source of light. Fluorescent lamp is not a point source of light. A point source is like a light from a distant star seen through a small telescope or light passing through a pinhole or other small aperture viewed from a distance much greater than the size of the hole.

2 CHAPTER

Prism

We have already discussed in Chapter 1 that when a ray of light strikes a medium of greater density at right angle to the direction of the separating surface, the ray does not change its path but its velocity is reduced and when it strikes a medium of lesser density its velocity is increased. However, when the same ray strikes a medium of different density obliquely, it deviates from its path. In other words, when a ray of light enters a denser medium from a rarer medium (e.g., from air to glass), it deviates towards normal and when it enters from denser to rarer medium (e.g., glass to air), it deviates away from normal.

PRISM

A *prism* is a refracting medium bound by two plane surfaces which are inclined at an angle called the apical angle or the refracting angle of the prism. When a ray of light passes through a prism it gets deviated towards its base according to Snell's Law. The image appears to be deviated towards its apex. It is virtual and erect. The angle of deviation is the angle between the incident ray and the emergent ray. Deviation is minimal when the light passes through the prism symmetrically, i.e., when the angle of incidence is equal to the angle of emergence. The angle of deviation of a prism = Half of the apical angle or angle of refraction. Thus a prism of refracting angle 10° (a 10° prism) deviates the light through 5° and has a power of 10 prism diopters.

Nomenclature of Prism

Apex

The point where the two refracting surfaces of prism meet. 'O' is the apex in **Figure 2.1**.

Base

The side of the prism opposite the apex is called the base of the prism. AB is the base in **Figure 2.1**.

Angle of Deviation

This is the angle formed between incident ray and the emergent ray. KCE is the angle of deviation in **Figure 2.1**.

Prism Diopter

It denotes power of prism. One prism diopter is that power of a prism which displaces the image of an object by one cm when object is placed at a distance of one meter from the prism.

Strength of a prism can also be expressed in degrees and centrads. Degree is concerned with apical angle.

$1° = 2$ prism diopters.

Centrad is that strength of a prism which produces a deviation of 1 cm of arc at a distance of 1 meter.

Apical Angle

It is also called the refracting angle. It is formed between the two refracting surfaces of prism. AOB is the apical angle in **Figure 2.1**.

Strength of a prism depends upon different factors namely the refractive index of prism material, angle of incidence and the apical

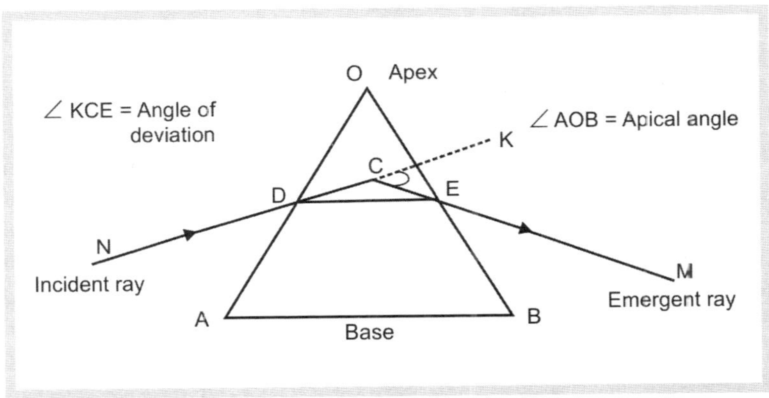

Fig. 2.1: Prism

angle of the prism. In thin prisms used in ophthalmic practice, angle of deviation is equal to half the apical angle of prism.

Uses

Diagnostic Uses

- Objective measurement of angle of deviation
- Measurement of fusional reserve
- Diagnosis of microtropia

Instruments

- Applanation tonometer
- Indirect ophthalmoscopes
- Keratometer
- Operating microscope
- Synoptophore
- Haidinger brushes

Therapeutic Uses

- Treatment of convergence insufficiency
- Treatment of diplopia

Miscellaneous Uses

- Low vision aids
- Hemianopic spectacles
- Recumbent spectacles

How to Detect and Measure Strength of a Prism?

Manual Method

See a straight line through a prism. It appears broken. Line appears to be deviated towards its apex **(Fig. 2.2)**. Now place a prism of known strength in such a way that base is towards apex of test prism. When prism of correct power is chosen, straight line appears unbroken again.

Another method of detecting prism clinically is that if a prism is rotated, the image of any object seen through it shows swinging movements.

With Lensometer?

Place a prism on the platform. Look through eyepiece of lensometer. The green target appears deviated. If you move the prism to bring the

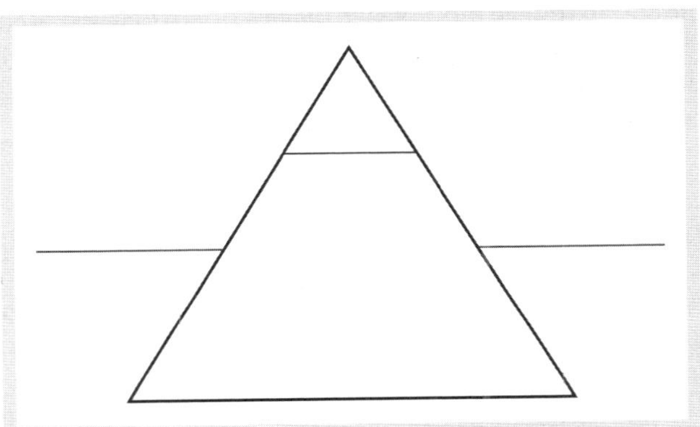

Fig. 2.2: Detection of prism *(A straight line appears broken through a prism and the broken part appears to be deviated towards apex of prism).*

target in the center, it cannot be brought in the center. This verifies that this is a prism. The target is deviated towards the apex of the prism.

Now combine a prism of known power with prism of unknown power placed apex to base. Place this combination on the platform and see through the lensometer. The target has moved towards the center. Choose the power of known prism by hit and trial method such that the combination makes the target move exactly in the center. This is the power of unknown prism, i.e., equal to the power of known prism.

Another Method

Check prism by using the Prism Reference Point (PRP), also called the Prism Compensation Device in the lensometer by noting the displacement of the mires from the central ring of the PRP. Each ring is marked with a number, the center is zero. Each ring represents one diopter of prism. If the mires are located two rings from the center, the prescription contains 2 diopters of prism.

Placement of a Prism

When a prism is used in eye, its position is indicated by its base; like base out, base in, base up, etc. Base out means that thicker side of prism is towards the temple. In **Figure 2.3** rays from an object O are not only falling on fovea of one eye but also extrafoveal point of other eye because that eye is convergent. Patient complains of confusion and diplopia. To relieve diplopia we place a prism of calculated power with base out (prism is placed with apex towards deviation), ray of light gets deviated towards base of prism and falls on fovea. Thus patient is relieved of diplopia.

Rotating Prism

When two prisms are placed apex to base, they behave like a thick plate of glass. If they are rotated in opposite directions, they produce the effect of a single prism with gradually increasing strength. The strength is maximum when they lie apex to apex and deviation of this combination of prisms is equal to the sum of the deviations of two prisms. Rotating prisms are used to overcome diplopia. One prism may be placed before one eye and the other before the other eye. Deviation is thus distributed equally between the two eyes.

COMPOUNDING AND RESOLVING PRISM POWERS

As we know that objects seen through a prism appear to be deviated towards its apex. Practically orientation of a prism is specified by writing the direction of its base, i.e., base up, down out and in. Base out and in means base is towards temple and nose respectively. Oblique prisms are specified by using 360° scale, e.g., base 40° means base up along 40° whereas base 230° means base down along 50°.

The process of adding prism powers together is known as compounding prism powers. If two prisms of power 2 and 3 prism

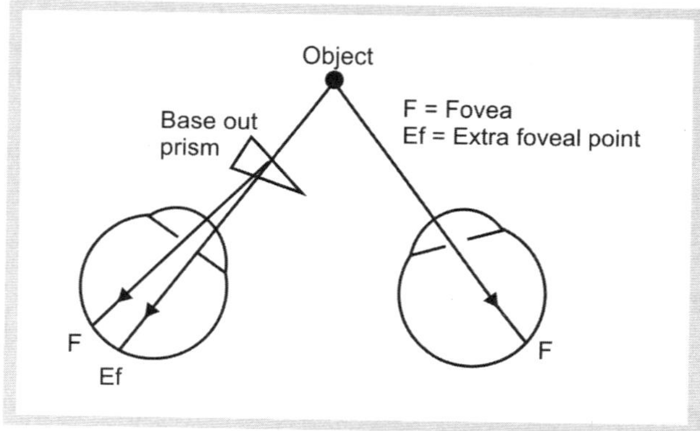

Fig. 2.3: Placement of prism.

diopters are prescribed with base in and out respectively, then it is simply prescription of prism 1 prism diopter base out.

If a prism is to be prescribed in horizontal and vertical meridians both, i.e., at right angles to each other, it can be prescribed as a single resultant prism by using Pythagoras theorem. Thus if a 3 prism diopter prism needs to be given with base up and 4 prism diopter prism base in, it can be prescribed as a single prism of 5 prism diopter at 37° for right eye.

Now if 5 prism diopter at 37° for right eye needs to be broken into its components, the process is known as resolving prism powers.

Refraction of Light

TRIAL SET

It is a box containing different types of spherical and cylindrical lenses along with prisms of different power, trial frame, cross cylinder and some other things like Maddox rod, stenopeic slit, pinhole, occluder, red-green glass, etc. **(Fig. 3.1)**.

Trial Frame

It is an adjustable frame meant to hold different kinds of lenses during retinoscopy and refraction of eye. It is designed in such a

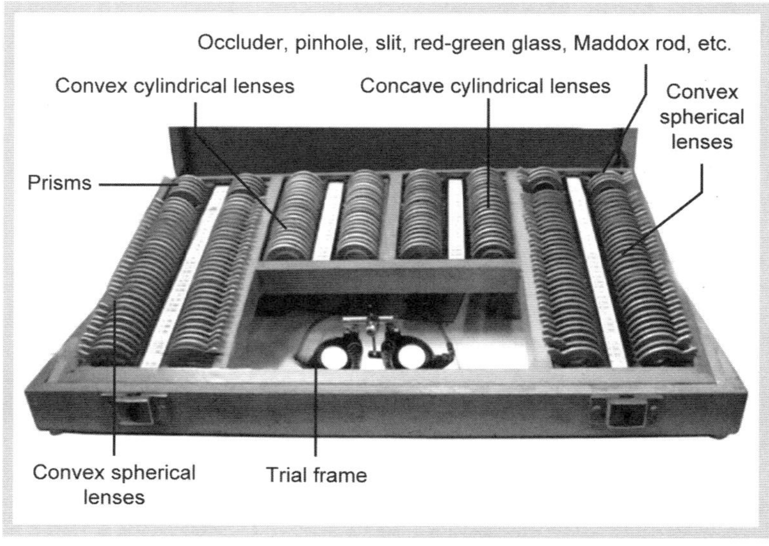

Fig. 3.1: Trial set (*For color version, see Plate 1*).

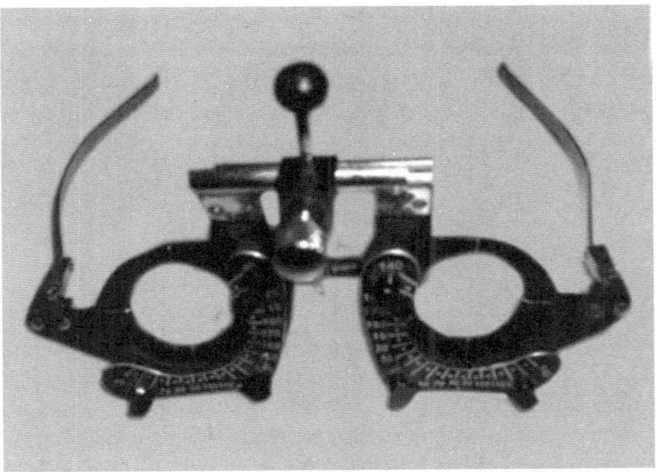

Fig. 3.2: Trial frame.

way that a combination of spherical lens and a cylindrical lens along with an occluder or pin hole can be placed in it simultaneously. Temple length and interpupillary distance can be adjusted as per requirements of the patient. Degree of axis is calibrated on both the rims of trial frame. Least number of lenses should be placed in the trial frame to create the desired power. Highest powered lens should be placed closest to the cornea (in the back lens clamp). Lenses should be replaced as quickly and accurately as possible **(Fig. 3.2)**.

Maddox Rod

It is used to detect and measure heterophoria (latent squint) for distance.

Technique

Patient is made to sit at a distance of 1 meter for smaller scale and 6 meters for bigger scale from tangent scale. He is asked to look at a point source of light with one eye and through a Maddox rod with other eye. A Maddox rod converts a point source of light into a streak. A normal person with no heterophoria (orthophoria) sees a bulb and a red streak passing through the center of the bulb. If a person is suffering from heterophoria, the red streak will pass from right side

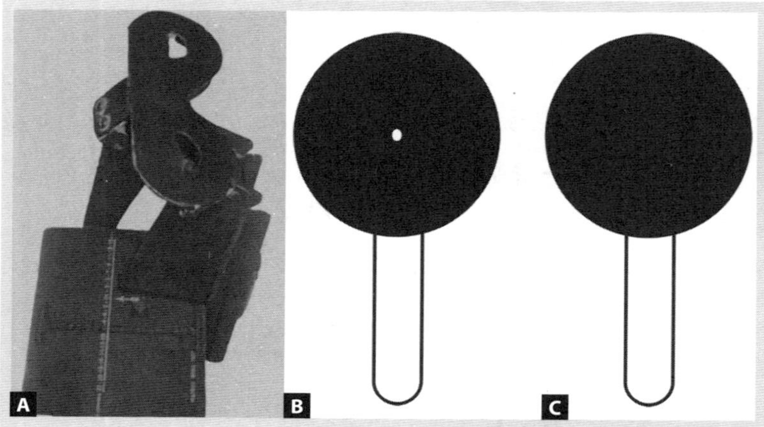

Figs. 3.3A to C: (A) Maddox wing; (B) Pinhole; (C) Occluder.

or left side or up and down side of bulb depending upon exophoria, esophoria, hyperphoria and hypophoria. *Heterophoria for near is detected with Maddox wing* **(Figs. 3.3A to C)**.

Principle

- Maddox rod breaks binocularity and latent squint becomes manifest.
- It is used to detect function of macula when media is not clear, e.g., before cataract surgery. A person with normal macular function sees a streak when he looks at a point source of light. This streak becomes broken if macula is not healthy.

Stenopeic Slit

- It is used to detect axis of astigmatism (*see* **Chapter 8**).
- It is used to differentiate between colored haloes of cataract and glaucoma. This test is known as Emsley Finscham Test. When we pass a slit from right to left in front of cornea, the colored halo due to cataract breaks but colored halo of glaucoma remains as such. This is because; in glaucoma colored halo is due to corneal edema which is homogeneous. In cataract, it is due to accumulation of water droplets in lens; which is a heterogeneous phenomenon.

Pinhole

It is like an occluder with a 1 mm hole in the center. In case of refractive error vision is improved with pinhole. However, if there is a central media opacity, use of pinhole decreases the visual acuity. If there is macular pathology, vision does not increase with use of pinhole **(Figs. 3.3A to C)**.

Pinhole Improves Vision in Case of Refractive Error. Why?

In case of refractive error, rays of light coming from infinity are focused either in front of retina (Myopia) or behind the retina (Hypermetropia) and a blur circle is formed on retina. Bigger is the size of blur circle, lesser is the visual acuity. With pinhole, size of blur circle is reduced and thus visual acuity improves as shown in **Figure 3.4**.

Occluder

It is used to occlude the eyeball for testing vision and doing refraction.

Red-Green Glass

- It is used for diplopia charting. Red glass is put before right eye and green before left eye by convention.
- It is also used for Worth's Four Dot test **(Fig. 3.5)**. This test is done to detect suppression and malingering (a person lies). Snellen's chart bears two green, one red and one white dot. Under normal conditions a person can see one red and one pink dot (two dots) with right eye using red glasses. With left eye using green glasses

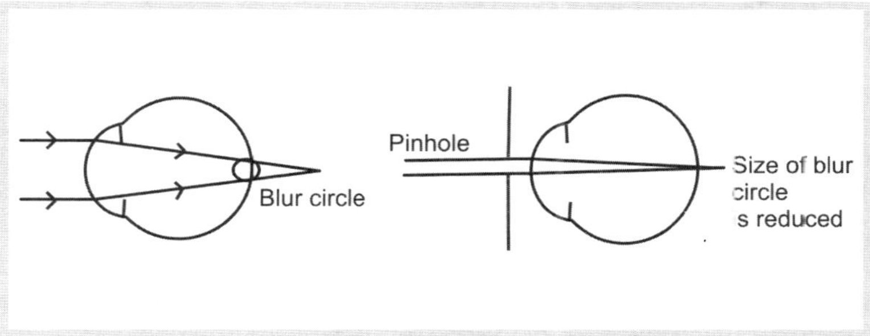

Fig. 3.4: Pinhole effect.

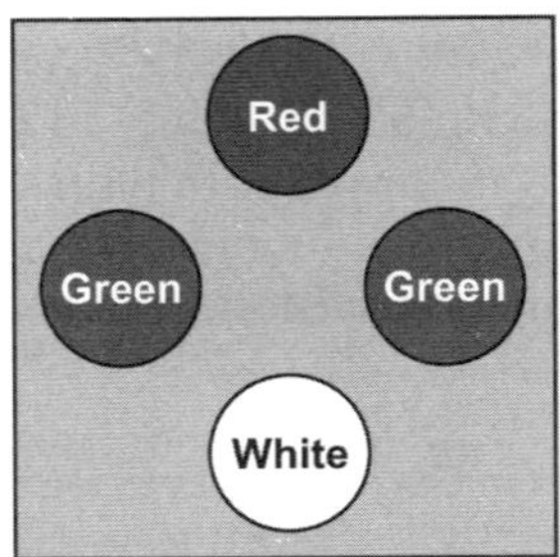

Fig. 3.5: Worth's four dot test (*For color version, see Plate 1*).

he can see two green and one light green dot (three dots). Red dot cannot be seen through green glass and vice versa as combination of red and green becomes black. Patient is asked to wear red glass in front of right eye and green glass in front of left eye. He is asked to tell how many dots he can see with right, left and both eyes separately.

The result is interpreted as below:

- *Right eye suppression*—three green dots seen with both eyes open.
- *Left eye suppression*—two red dots with both eyes open.
- *Normal person*—four dots with both eyes open.
- *Malingerer*—Wavering answers.
- *A person having diplopia*—five dots, two red with right eye and three green with left eye.

Prisms of different powers from 1 to 10 prism diopters are there in the trial set.

Spherical and Cylindrical Lenses

Different powers of convex and concave lenses ranging from 0.25 DS to 20.00 DS and 0.25 DC to 6.00 DC are available in pairs in the trial set.

Lens and its Types

A lens is a transparent medium bound by two surfaces which are part of spheres. Lenses are basically of two types: convex and concave.

A convex lens may be biconvex, plano-convex and concavo-convex or convex meniscus lens. Similarly a concave lens may be biconcave, plano-concave and convexo-concave or concave meniscus **(Fig. 3.6)**.

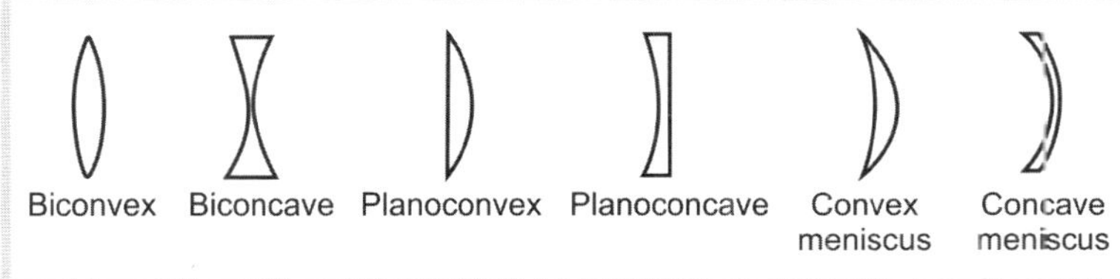

Fig. 3.6: Different types of lenses.

A convex lens is considered as collection of prisms placed base to base and a concave lens is considered as collection of prisms placed apex to apex.

A convex lens is a converging lens and a concave lens is a diverging lens. Why?

A convex lens is made up of prisms placed base to base and a concave lens is made up of prisms placed apex to apex. We know that power of a prism is maximum at its apex and minimum at its base. At the same time a ray, which strikes the prism obliquely, gets deviated towards its base **(Figs. 3.7 and 3.8)**.

Notations of a Lens

- **Principal axis:** It is a line that represents a ray of light which passes through the lens undeviated.
- **Optical center:** It is that point in the lens through which the ray of light passes undeviated.

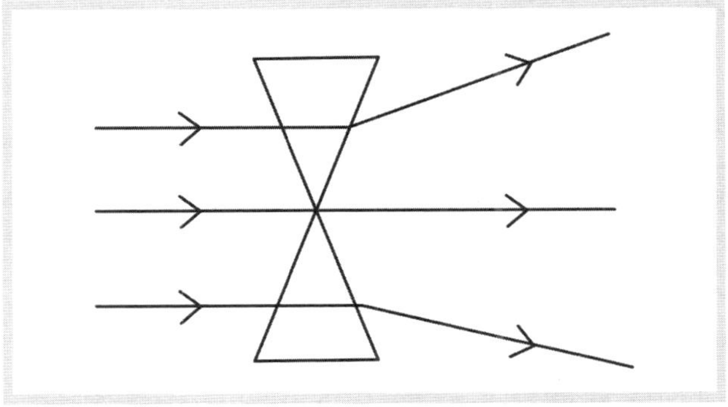

Fig. 3.7: Concave lens diverges rays of light.

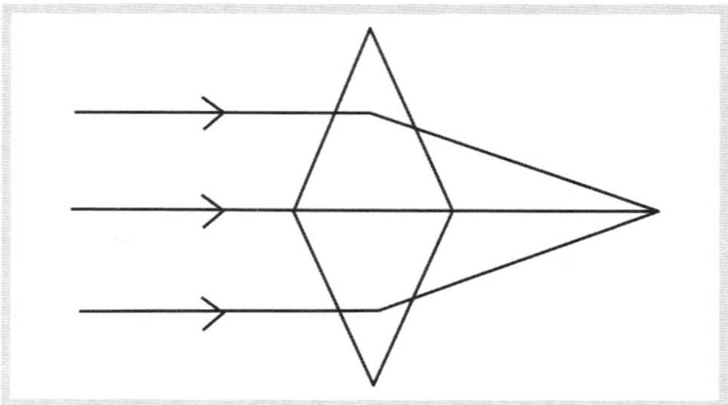

Fig. 3.8: Convex lens converges rays of light.

- **Focus:** It is that point on the principal axis of a lens where the parallel rays of light coming from infinity after passing through the lens get focused in case of a convex lens or appear to come from in case of a concave lens.
- **First principal focus** (F_1 in **Fig. 3.9**): It is a point on the principal axis of a lens such that the rays of light starting from this point in a convex lens or appearing to meet at this point in a concave lens become parallel to principal axis after refraction from the lens.
- **Second principal focus** (F_2 in **Fig. 3.9**): It is point on the principal axis such that the rays of light coming from infinity and hence running parallel to principal axis pass through this point in a convex lens and appear to come from this point in a concave lens.

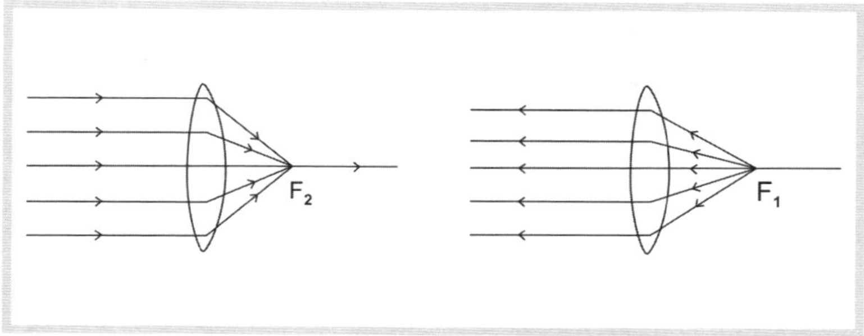

Fig. 3.9: First and second principal focus.

- **Center of curvature:** It is the center of curvature of the sphere of which lens is a part.
- **Focal length:** This is the distance between optical center of a lens and the focus.
- **Diopter:** It is the unit of measurement of power of a lens. It is denoted by abbreviation D. One diopter power corresponds to a lens of one meter focal length. Power of lens is inversely proportional to focal length, i.e.,

$$D = \frac{\text{d}}{F\,(\text{in meters})}$$

- **Back vertex power:** The effective power of a lens measured from the surface towards the eye is known as the back vertex power of lens. The distance between the back surface of spectacle lens and front surface of cornea is known as back vertex distance. If this back vertex distance changes, the back vertex power or effective power of lens also changes.
- **Depth of focus:** The greatest distance through which an object point can be moved without spoiling the image is termed as the depth of focus. As the size of aperture of optical system increases, the depth of focus decreases. Thus, as the size of pupil increases the depth of focus decreases. Hence, depth of focus is increased during accommodation.

Image Formation by a Convex Lens (Fig. 3.10)

Sl. No.	*Position of object*	*Characteristics of image*
1.	At infinity	Image is formed at focus on opposite side of lens, pinpoint size and real
2.	Away from 2f	Image is formed between f and 2f on opposite side, real, inverted and smaller in size as compared to size of object
3.	At center of curvature	Image is formed at 2f on opposite side, real, inverted and equal in size as that of object
4.	Between f and 2f	Image is formed away from 2f on opposite side, real, inverted and bigger in size as compared to size of object
5.	At focus	Image is formed at infinity, real and magnified
6.	Between f and optical center of a lens	Virtual, magnified and erect image is formed on the same side of the lens

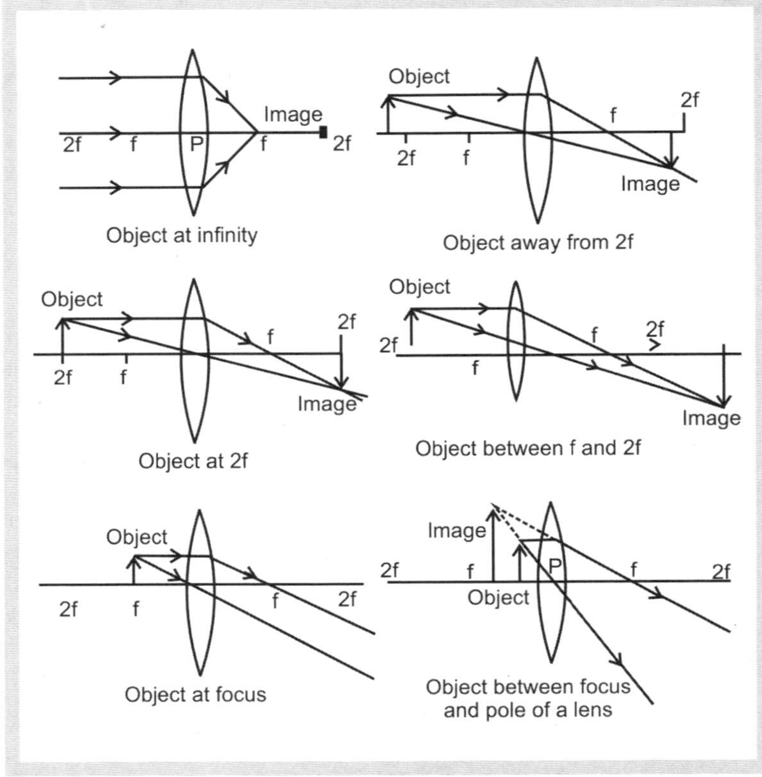

Fig. 3.10: Image formation by a convex lens.

- **Image formation by a concave lens:** Rays coming from infinity are diverged by a concave lens. The image produced is always virtual, minified, and erect and on the same side of the lens whatever may be the position of the object **(Fig. 3.11)**.
- **Cylindrical lens:** A cylindrical lens is a segment of the cylinder cut parallel to its axis. These lenses do not have same curvature in all meridians. Axis of a cylindrical lens is parallel to that of a cylinder of which it is a segment. In simple words, a cylindrical lens has no power in the direction of its axis but behaves like a spherical lens in a direction at right angles to its axis.

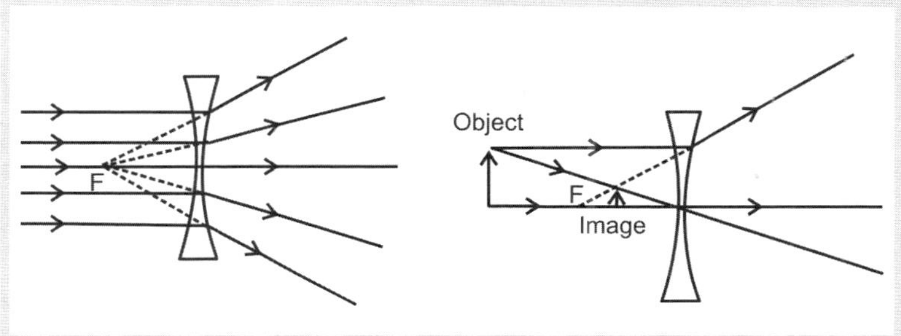

Fig. 3.11: Image formation by a concave lens.

Uses of Lens

- A convex lens is used to correct presbyopia, and hypermetropia.
- It is used as a magnifying lens to see details of an object. It is also used in low vision aids. It is also used in various types of ophthalmic instruments like microscopes, slit lamps, ophthalmoscopes, etc.
- A concave lens is used to correct myopia. It is also used in ophthalmoscopes and as Hruby lens.

Identification of a Lens

Sl. No.	*Convex lens*	*Concave lens*
1.	It is thick in the center and thin at margins	It is thin in the center and thick at margins
2.	Convex lens is a magnifying lens, objects appear bigger in size	It is a minifying lens, objects appear smaller in size
3.	If we move a lens, the image moves in opposite direction	If we move a lens, the image moves in same direction
4.	It is denoted by PLUS (+) sign	It is denoted by MINUS (–) sign
5.	It is used to correct hypermetropia and presbyopia	It is used to correct myopia

Both convex and concave lenses are of two types:

Sl. No.	*Spherical lens*	*Cylindrical lens*
1.	Movement of image can be seen in all directions	Movement of image can be seen only in one direction, i.e., at right angle to its axis. There is no movement of image along the axis of lens
2.	If we rotate a lens, there is no distortion of image	If we rotate a lens, there is distortion of image

Compound Lens

It is a combination of spherical and cylindrical lens. If we move a compound lens, the image moves in all directions (due to spherical power). At the same time if lens is rotated, the image shows distortion (due to cylindrical power).

COMBINATION OF LENSES

If two thin lenses are placed in contact with each other in such a way that their optical axes coincides with each other (homocentric system of lenses) the net power of the combination of lenses will be given by the algebraic sum of the power of two lenses. However, if the two lenses are separated together by a distance (d) the net power of combination of lenses (f) is given by: $\frac{1}{f} = \frac{1}{f_2} + \frac{1}{f_{1-d}}$ where f_1 is the focal length of lens no 1 and f_2 is the focal length of lens no 2 and d is the distance between two lenses in meters **(Fig. 3.12)**.

Combination of Cylindrical Lenses (Fig. 3.13)

- If two cylindrical lenses are placed in contact with each other with their axis parallel to each other, the net power of the lenses will be the algebraic sum of the power of two cylinders.
- If their axis is at right angle to each other, the net power of the lenses will depend upon:
  - If they are either concave or convex with equal power—the combination will behave as a spherical lens with same sign.
  - If their sign is same but power is different—the combination will behave as a compound lens.

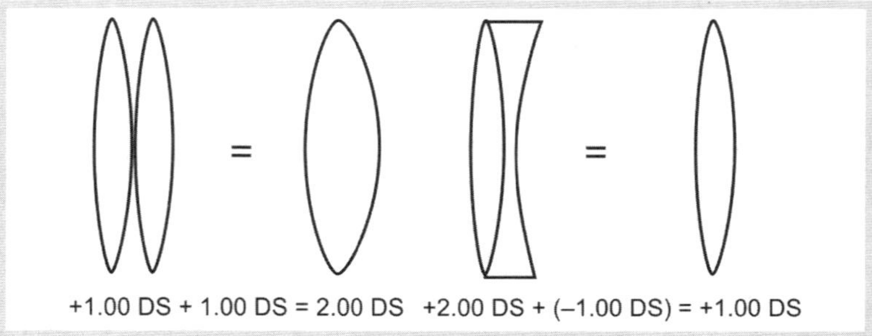

Fig. 3.12: Combination of spherical lenses.

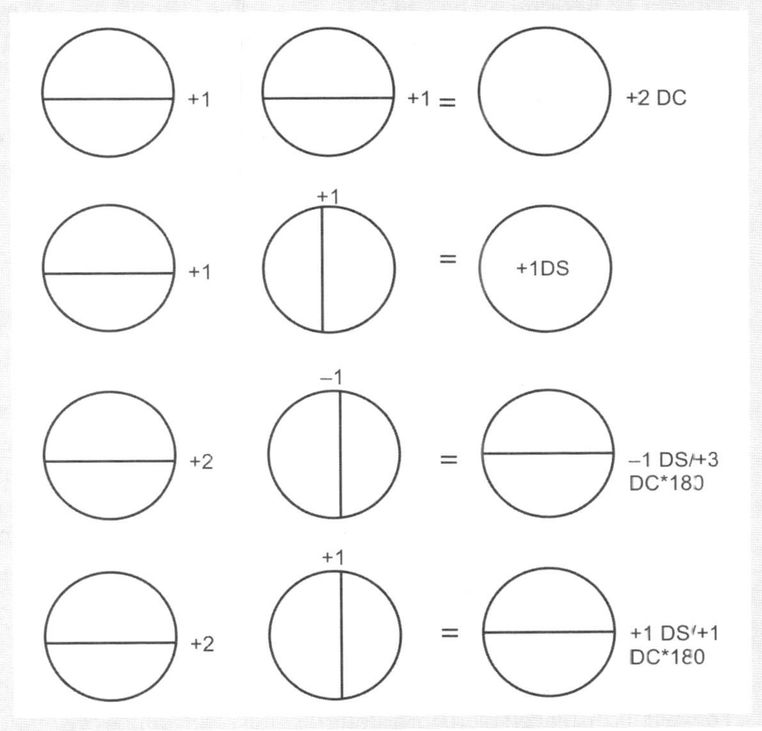

Fig. 3.13: Combination of cylindrical lenses.

- If their sign is different and power is same/different, it will behave as a cross compound lens, i.e., a combination of lens in which power of cylinder is more than power of spherical lens with opposite signs.

Decentration of Lenses and Prismatic Effect

When we wear spectacles the visual axis of eyeball must pass through the optical center of lenses. If it does not happen it introduces prismatic effect. If prismatic effect is small it may go unnoticed but if it is a marked decentration, patient complains of eyestrain symptoms. The following general principles should be kept in mind regarding decentration of lenses:

- 1.00 D *spherical lens* gives 1 diopter prismatic effect if decentered by 10 mm. Similarly, a +10 D spherical lens gives prismatic effect of

1 diopter if decentered by 1 mm. This example clearly shows how important is marking of optical center while fitting of glasses in high power lenses. The dioptric strength of the prism is calculated by the following formula:

$$\Delta = C \times D$$

Where Δ = Prismatic effect in prism diopters
C = Decentration in CM
D = Power of lens in diopters

- Decentration of a *cylindrical lens* in its axis produces no prismatic effect. Decentration of a cylinder at right angle to its axis produces the same prismatic effect as produced by a spherical lens, i.e., 1.00 D cylindrical lens if decentered by 1 cm at right angle to its axis; produces prismatic effect of one prism diopter.
- If a *compound lens* is decentered, it produces prismatic effect of a spherical lens along its axis and algebraic sum of prismatic effect produced by spherical and cylindrical lens if decentered at right angles to its axis, e.g., if a +2.00 DS/+1.00 DC × 180° lens is decentered by 1 cm along 180° it produces prismatic effect of two prism diopters but if decentered along 90°, it produces prismatic effect of three prism diopters.
- If it is a *cross compound lens,* i.e., the power of cylinder is more than the power of sphere with opposite sign, the decentration produces prismatic effect as below: Suppose a prescription of +2.00 DS/–3.00 DC × 90° is displaced by 10 mm along 90°, it will introduce prismatic effect of 2 prism diopters but if it is displaced by 10 mm along 180°, it will introduce prismatic effect of 1 prism diopter (+2 – 3 = –1). Here it is to be kept in mind that a convex lens if displaced downwards or outwards, it is just like prescribing prism with base down or base out respectively. Similarly if a concave lens is displaced downwards or outwards, it is like prescribing a prism with base up or in respectively, i.e., the convex and concave lenses have opposite effect.
- If decentration is required in both horizontal and vertical meridians, it is produced in oblique meridian.

Clinical Applications of Decentration

Decentration has certain desirable effects also in clinical practice.

- In lenses for near vision the optical center is displaced inward by 2.5 mm and downward by 6.5 mm on an average so that the optical center coincides with the visual axis.

- In order to adapt glasses for an asymmetrical face. Suppose a patient has left eye displaced downwards as compared to right eye due to some congenital abnormality. A pair of spectacles with left rim down and right rim up appears cosmetically unacceptable. So lens of left rim can be decentered down so that the visual axis passes through the optical center of glass and there is no prismatic effect.
- To treat diplopia due to exophoria, esophoria, hyperphoria, etc.
- To augment exercises for heterophoria.

Prentice Rule

It is a formula used to prescribe prism by decentering the lens. It states that: P = cf; where
P = Prism diopters
c = Decentration in cm
f = Power of lens

Clinical Applications

Sometimes instead of grinding prism into the lens, the lens is decentered to obtain prismatic effect. Thus the weight and the cost of the glass, both can be reduced.

How to Check Power of Unknown Lens?

It is by two methods:

1. **Neutralization method:** Take a lens of known power with opposite sign. Place the two lenses together and note movement of image with movement of combination of lenses. Increase or decrease the power of known lens till the combination of lenses does not show any movement. Note down the power of known lens. This is also the power of unknown lens with opposite sign.
   During neutralization always keep the lens close to the eyeball and see an object, which is far off so that minimal movement of image in case of small power lens can be easily appreciated.
2. **Lensometer and Auto-lensometer (Figs. 3.14 to 3.16):** It is also known as Focimeter or Vertex refractionometer.

Lensometer is based on the principle that image of a target; which is usually a ring of dotted circle, is focused by a standard lens when seen through a telescope. When an unknown lens is inserted into

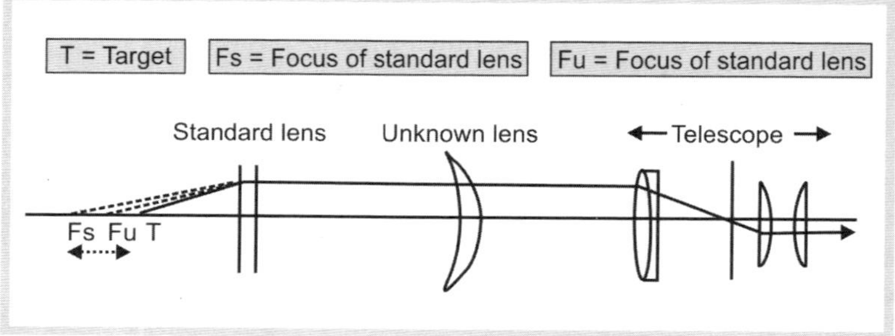

Fig. 3.14: Optics of lensometer.

this optical system the position of target is changed. The excursion required to bring target back into focus is directly proportional to the back vertex power of lens **(Fig. 3.14)**.

First of all when instrument is calibrated the emerging rays are parallel and image of target T is seen at the focal point of standard lens Fs. When unknown lens is placed between the standard lens and the telescope with its back surface facing the standard lens, the image of target T becomes blurred because it is formed at focal point of unknown lens and the emergent rays are no more parallel.

In order to see clear image of target T knob has to be rotated so that the emergent rays again become parallel. The amount of knob rotated to focus the target is directly proportional to the strength of unknown lens which can be directly read from the scale.

How to Use?

First of all the instrument should be calibrated. Focus the scale with eyepiece. Focus the green colored target with knob. Target is seen as a circle of dots. Note down the reading. It should be zero. Now place the lens with unknown power on the platform of lensometer. Adjust the knob to refocus the target. Take fresh reading. This gives the power of unknown lens.

In case of a cylindrical lens after focusing the target, axis of target should also be noted. This is the axis of the unknown lens. If the unknown lens is a spherical one, the green colored target is seen as circle of dots. If it is a cylindrical or compound lens the dots become a series of lines. The length of lines is directly proportional to the power of the cylinder.

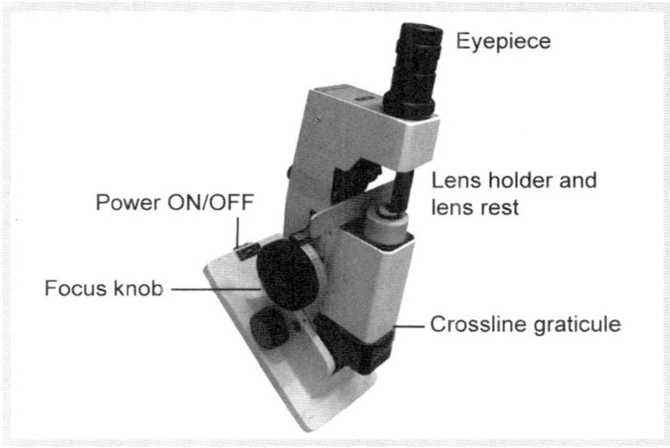

Fig. 3.15: Lensometer.

In case of a compound lens after placing the lens, the target is focused and reading taken. Here the target is focused in form of series of lines with some particular direction. This is the power of spherical component. Now refocus the target. Now the direction of lines is at right angles to the previous direction. Now take second reading. The difference between the first and second readings is the power of the cylindrical component. The axis shown at second reading is the axis of the cylinder. In simple words:

- First reading = Power of spherical
- Second reading—First reading = Power of cylinder
- Axis of the second reading = Axis of cylinder.

Uses of Lensometer

- To check the power of unknown lens
- To check the axis of unknown lens
- To mark axis of unknown lens
- To check and mark optical center of a lens
- To detect and measure power of unknown prism

Manual lensometers are of two types. Projection lensometer in which many persons can see reading at one time and there is no need to adjust the eyepiece. The other design is the eyepiece lensometer in which only one person can see the reading at one time and eyepiece needs to be adjusted every time.

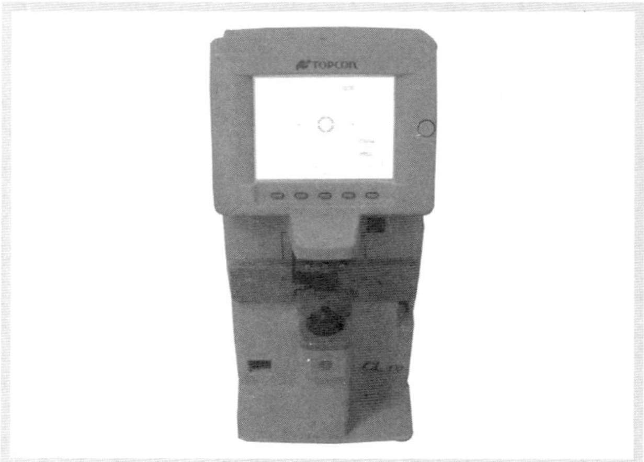

Fig. 3.16: Auto-lensometer.

Sources of Error

- If eyepiece is not adjusted prior to putting the lens on platform. 0.25 D error can creep in by this mistake.
- If calibration of instrument is not done.
- If there is a lag in the movement of knob.
- If focusing of target is not done properly.
- If reading is not taken properly. Ideally our eyes should be at the same level as the level of the scale to avoid error.

How to Mark Axis of a Cylinder with Lensometer?

Place the lens on platform (lens rest). Rotate the lens in such a way that its axis becomes 180° as seen through eyepiece. Now put some ink or marker in the slot provided on lensometer for marking axis. Press the knob to mark on the lens. Three points are marked on lens in this way. Join these three points; this marks the axis of the cylinder. The central point is the optical center of the lens.

Effectivity of Lens

If a concave lens is moved away from eyeball or a convex lens is moved towards eyeball, its effectivity decreases.

If a concave lens is moved towards eyeball or a convex lens is moved away from eyeball, its effectivity increases **(Fig. 3.17)**.

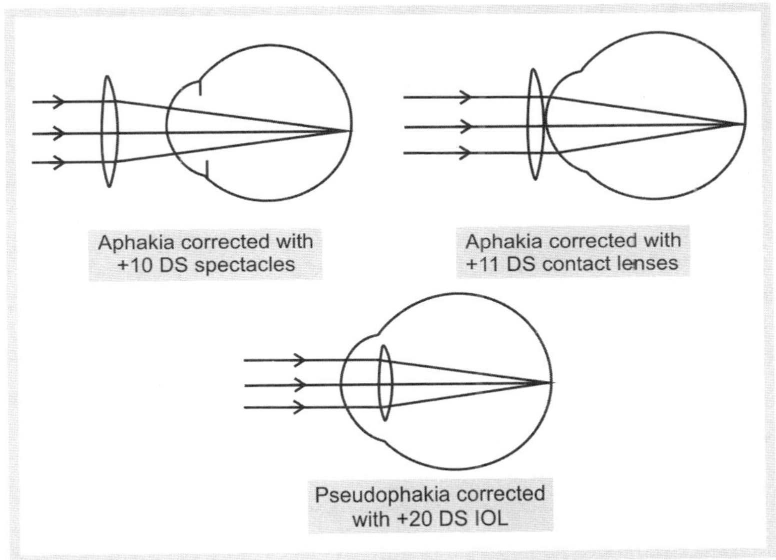

Fig. 3.17: Change in position of lens produces change in effectivity of lens.

Examples

If a minus 10 DS spectacles needs to be replaced with contact lens, its power has to be decreased to –9 DS because when a concave lens (in form of spectacle) is displaced posteriorly (in form of contact lens) its effective power is increased and to achieve emmetropia its power has to be decreased from –10 DS to –9 DS.

During cataract surgery, crystalline lens of eyeball is replaced with plus 20 DS IOL. If IOL is not implanted and patient is prescribed glasses, its power would be around plus 10 DS. This is because when plus lens (in form of IOL) is displaced anteriorly (in form of spectacles), its effective power is increased and to achieve emmetropia its power has to be decreased.

Change in position of lens produces change in retinal image size: If a convex lens is moved away from eyeball (anterior principal focus) or a concave lens is moved towards eyeball the size of retinal image is increased. If a concave lens is moved away from eyeball (anterior principal focus) or a convex lens is moved towards eyeball the size of retinal image is decreased **(Fig. 3.18)**.

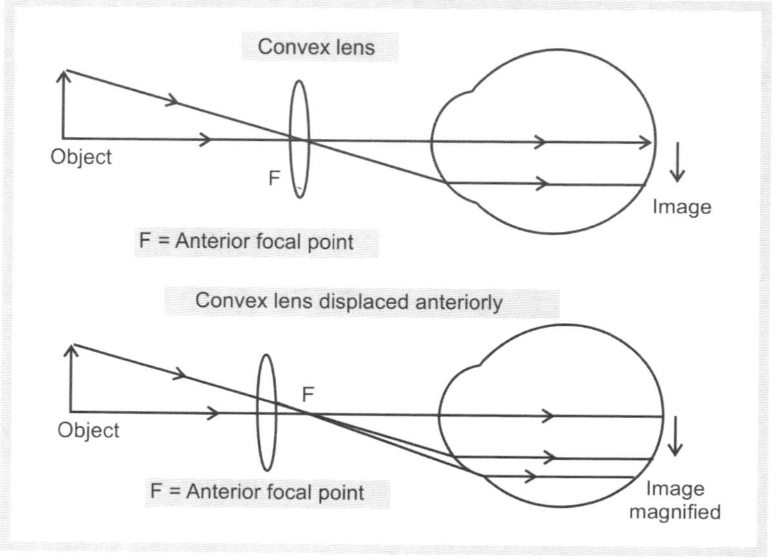

Fig. 3.18: Change in position of lens produces change in retinal image size.

This is the reason that a patient with aphakic glasses experiences 30% magnification of image, with contact lens 5–6% and with IOL only 1% magnification of image.

OPTICS OF THE EYE

Human eyeball is compared with a camera. Iris acts as shutter and retina acts as negative film. The refracting components of eyeball namely cornea, lens, aq. humor and vitreous humor are compared with lens of the camera. All these components form a homocentric system of lenses. Thus eyeball acts as a very strong convex lens with power of +60 D, cornea contributing +42 D and lens +18 D.

Gauss Theorem

Now eye can be considered as a homocentric system of so many lenses and calculation of power of the whole system becomes very tedious. A simple method of calculation was devised by Gauss popularly known as Gauss Theorem. He said that homocentric system of lenses can be treated as a whole if the object and image distances are measured from two theoretical planes called principal planes. The whole system can be resolved into six cardinal points:

- Two principal planes
- Two nodal points
- Two principal foci

According to Gauss concept, the cardinal data of schematic eye is as follows:

- Total dioptric power of eyeball is +60 D with lens contributing +18 D and cornea +42 D.
- The principal foci lie 15.7 mm in front of and 24.4 mm behind the cornea respectively.
- The cardinal points lie in the AC 1.35 mm and 1.60 mm behind the anterior surface of cornea respectively.
- The nodal points lie in the posterior part of lens 7.08 mm and 7.33 mm behind the anterior surface of cornea respectively.

The Reduced Eye

To simplify, the cardinal data listing has chosen single principal point and single nodal point. This is called Listing's Reduced Eye. He presented the following data:

- Total dioptric power of eyeball is +60 D.
- The principal point lies 1.5 mm behind the anterior surface of cornea.
- The nodal point is situated 7.2 mm behind the anterior surface of cornea.
- The anterior focal point is 15.7 mm in front of the anterior surface of cornea.
- The posterior focal point is 24.4 mm behind the anterior surface of cornea.
- The anterior focal length is 17.2 mm and the posterior focal length is 22.9 mm.

Donder further simplified the data treating eye as a single curved surface. According to him total dioptric power of eyeball is +60 D. Refractive index is taken as 1.33. Anterior and posterior focal length is taken as 15 mm and 20 mm, respectively. The plane of the curved surface is 2 mm behind the cornea with a radius of curvature of 5 mm. Nodal point is situated 5 mm behind the plane.

OPTICAL ABERRATIONS OF LENSES AND EYEBALL

Human eyeball is not a perfect optical system. There are certain optical aberrations which limit the definition of retinal image.

Spherical Aberration

Rays of light passing from central part of a lens come to a focus that is slightly away from the point where the peripheral rays are focused. This is because peripheral part of a lens has more power than the central part of a lens. Due to this phenomenon definition of retinal image becomes limited. In a convex lens peripheral rays are focused before the central rays. This is called *Positive Spherical Aberration.* In a concave lens, central rays are focused before the peripheral rays. This is called the *Negative Spherical Aberration* **(Fig. 3.19)**.

This phenomenon is little evident in our eyes. This is because nature has tried to neutralize the effect of spherical aberration by:

- Providing iris which cuts off the peripheral rays, thus only central part of lens is used for seeing. When we dilate the pupil spherical aberration becomes more evident and patient complains of blurring of vision.
- Making the peripheral part of cornea flatter than central part of cornea. This tries to neutralize the effect of aberration produced by lens.
- Central part of lens (nucleus) is more densely packed hence more refractive index than the peripheral part of lens.

The spectacle glasses normally used also have this optical defect. However glasses are available in the markets which are *aspheric or*

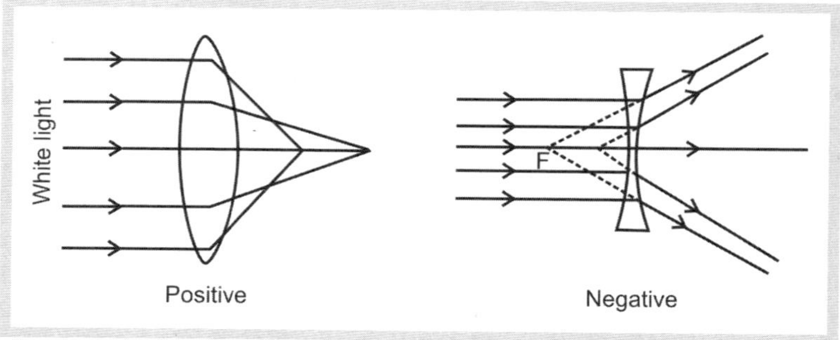

Fig. 3.19: Spherical aberration.

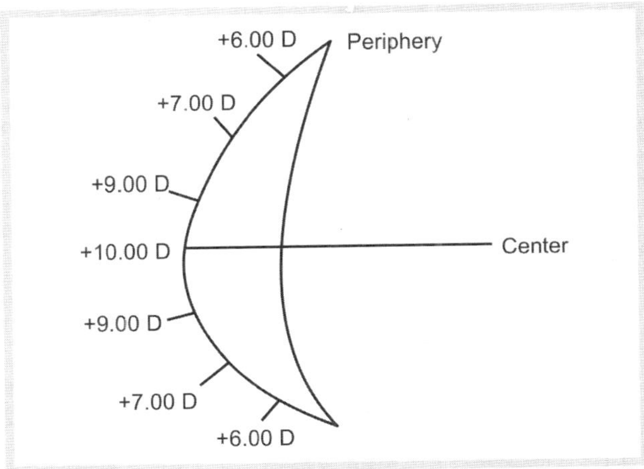

Fig. 3.20: Aspheric lens + 10.00 DSph.

aplanatic but they are costly. Such glasses are grinded in such a way that their curvature (and hence power) is maximum in the center and gradually decreases towards periphery. Thus an aspheric lens of +10 DS has a power of +10 DS at the center and +6 DS at the extreme periphery **(Fig. 3.20)**.

Chromatic Aberration

White light is made up of seven colors. Each color has different wavelength and thus suffer different deviation when passed through a lens. Thus red light suffers minimum deviation from its path and violet light suffers maximum deviation. A spectrum remembered by VIBGYOR is produced. Thus this effect also compromises the definition of retinal image. It also increases with increase in size of pupil. Thus a normal eye is myopic for violet light, emmetropic for yellow light and hypermetropic for red light. Thus to an emmetropic patient both violet and red lights appear equally sharp. This forms the basis of duochrome test **(Fig. 3.21)**.

An achromatic lens can be manufactured by combining two glasses of different dispersive power and different refractive index. Flint glass has a refractive index of 1.65 but dispersive power double than that of crown glass. Ref. index of crown glass is 1.5. Thus if a +2.00 DS lens of crown glass with +2d dispersive power is combined

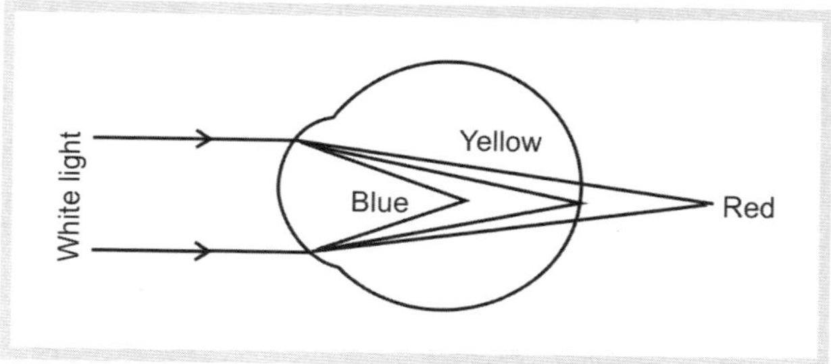

Fig. 3.21: Chromatic aberration.

with –1.00 DS lens of flint glass which has –2d dispersive power, a +1.00 DS lens with zero dispersive power is obtained **(Fig. 3.22)**.

Diffraction

When a bundle of rays of light travels through space, the peripheral rays tend to deviate away from the center. In simple language, this is because they do not have peripheral support. This effect is more if the bundle is narrow thus in a normal size pupil this aberration is more evident. As the size of pupil increases, diffraction of light decreases. Thus different bundles of ray when pass through a lens do not come to one focus but form concentric rings. Thus definition of image is compromised.

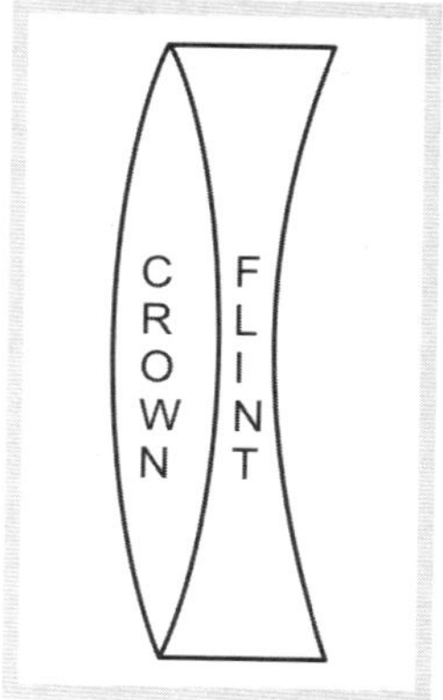

Fig. 3.22: Achromatic doublet.

Peripheral Aberrations

Certain phenomenon like *coma, oblique astigmatism and distortion of image* tend to make the image formed on peripheral part of retina less clearly defined. But they have little significance due to a peculiar shape of eyeball.

Coma is an aberration which affects light rays falling obliquely on the lens. Thus rays passing through different parts of lens are focused at different points and image formed is like shape of a coma. It may be positive or negative. Aplanatic lens can be used to get rid of this defect.

When rays of light fall obliquely on spherical lenses, they give rise to oblique astigmatism. This is because spherical lenses show different power in different meridians if rays fall obliquely on them.

When a grid pattern is observed through a high plus or high minus lens, the image appears distorted as seen in **Figure. 3.23.** This is called distortion. High power convex lens shows pincushion distortion as seen by a person using aphakic glasses and high minus lens shows barrel distortion.

All these types of aberrations can be measured by a test called aberrometry. This has a clinical application in doing LASIK laser surgery and making of intraocular lenses.

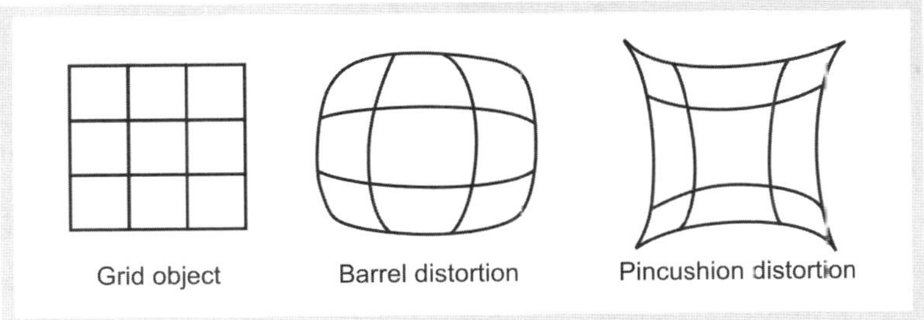

Fig. 3.23: Distortions.

4

CHAPTER

Reflection of Light

MIRROR

A mirror is a part of a hollow sphere whose one side is polished. Mirrors are of two types:

1. Plane mirror
2. Curved mirror

Plane Mirror

Image formed by a plane mirror is of the same size as the object, laterally inverted (right side appears towards left and left side appears towards right), virtual, erect and lies at the same distance behind the mirror as the object is in front **(Fig. 4.1A)**.

Curved Mirror

It can be of two types: Concave and Convex mirror. Concave mirror converges parallel rays of light and convex mirror diverges parallel rays of light. This is in contrast to concave lens which diverges parallel rays of light and convex lens which converges parallel rays of light **(Figs. 4.1B and 4.2)**. *Center of curvature and radius of curvature* of a spherical mirror are respectively the center and radius of the sphere of which the mirror was a part. *Pole* of the mirror is the geometric center of the reflecting surface.

The *principal axis* of the mirror is the line joining the pole to the center of curvature. *Principal focus* of a concave mirror is the point on the principal axis where the rays of light traveling parallel to the principal axis get focused after reflection. In convex mirror, these rays appear to meet but do not meet actually. That is why convex mirror always gives virtual image. These images are always erect and smaller than the size of the object **(Fig. 4.1B)**. Characteristics

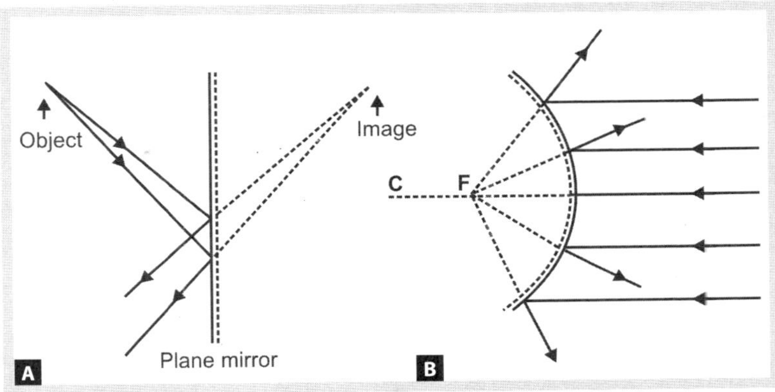

Figs. 4.1A and B: Virtual image formed by plane and convex mirrors.

of image formed by a concave mirror depend on the position of the object in relation to the mirror. If the object is between infinity and the principal focus, the image formed is real and inverted. If the object is between the pole and the principal focus, the image is virtual, erect and magnified **(Fig. 4.3)**. *Focal length* of the concave or convex mirror is the distance between the pole and the principal focus of the mirror. It is equal to half the radius of curvature, i.e., F = CP/2

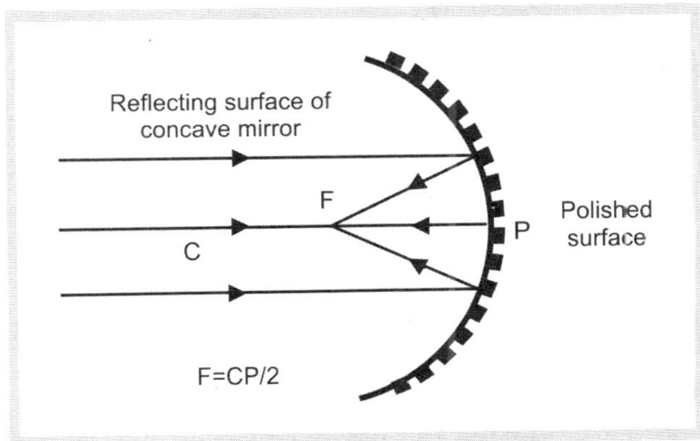

Fig. 4.2: Curved (concave) mirror.

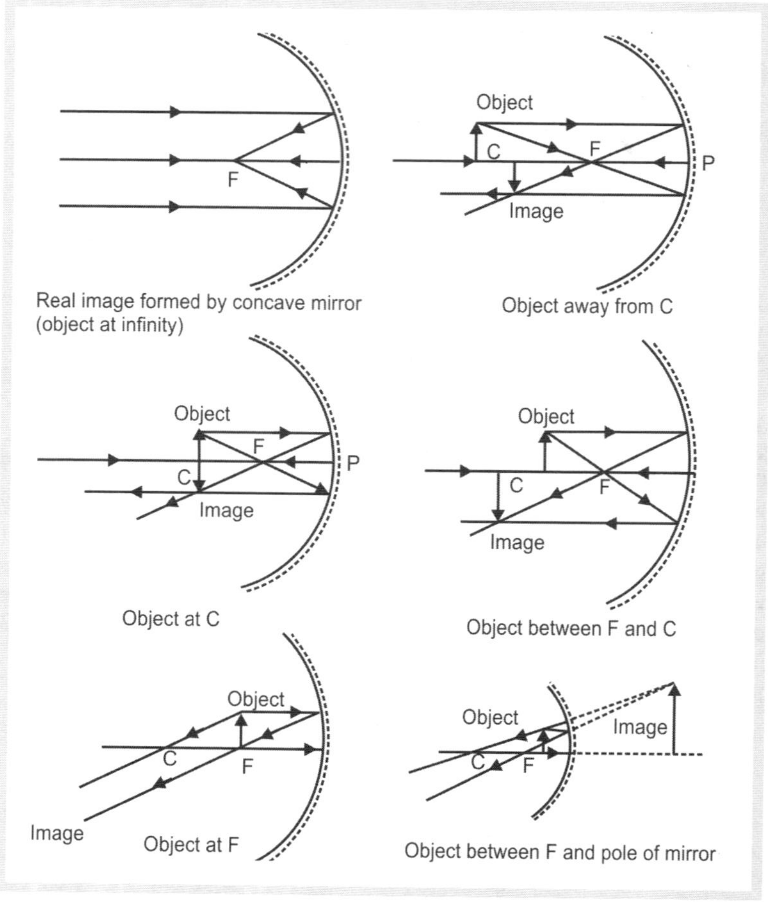

Fig. 4.3: Image formation by a concave mirror.

Uses of Concave Mirror

- Concave mirrors are used as reflectors in torchlights, film projectors, and searchlights.
- They are also used in telescopes.
- ENT specialists and dentists use concave mirror as light focusing device.
- Concave mirrors are is also used for retinoscopy in hazy media.

- They are also used as magnifiers.
- Solar cookers use concave mirror to focus sunlight.
- They are also used as shaving mirrors. When the face is kept between the mirror and its focus, its image is magnified and erect.

Uses of Convex Mirror

- They are used as rearview mirrors in vehicles. The image formed by this mirror is minified and erect, hence bigger area is visible.
- They are mounted on corners inside and outside the buildings where corridors and hallways intersect so as to avoid collisions.
- They are helpful to security personnel to keep a watch on larger area. Mirrors can be coated and cameras can be mounted inside.
- They are also used to inspect area difficult to get to. Convex mirror can be mounted on a rod with light and can be extended underside the object.

Image formed by a convex mirror is always virtual, minified and erect irrespective of the position of object.

A *real image* is one which is formed by *actual meeting of light rays* as occurs in concave mirror and convex lens. A *virtual image* is one in which *rays of light do not actually meet but appear to come from that point* as occurs in convex mirror and concave lens.

Images Formed by a Concave Mirror

Sl. No.	*Position of object*	*Characteristics of Image formed by concave mirror (Fig. 4.3)*
1.	At infinity	Image is formed at focus, pinpoint size and real
2.	Away from C	Image is formed between F and C, real, inverted and smaller in size as compared to size of object
3.	At center of curvature	Image is formed at C, real, inverted and equal in size as that of object
4.	Between F and C	Image is formed away from C, real, inverted and bigger in size as compared to size of object
5.	At focus	Image is formed at infinity, real and magnified
6.	Between F and pole of mirror	Virtual, magnified and erect image is formed behind the mirror

5
CHAPTER

Visual Angles and Axes of Eye

AXES AND ANGLES OF EYEBALL

Optical Axis

A line passing through center of cornea, center of lens and posterior pole of retina is the optical axis of eyeball **(ONA in Fig. 5.1)**.

Visual Axis

A line joining point of fixation with fovea and passing through nodal point of eyeball is called visual axis. The nodal point of eyeball is just anterior to posterior capsule of lens. Fixation point is the point which is being seen with fovea at any particular moment **(VNF in Fig. 5.1)**.

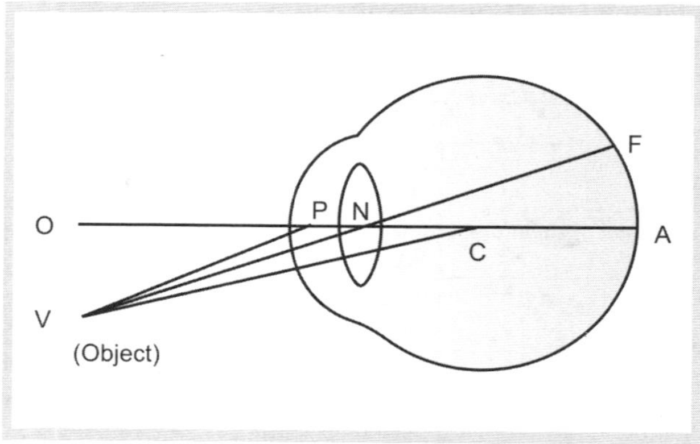

Fig. 5.1: Axes of eyeball.

Pupillary Axis

This is a straight line that passes through center of pupil **(OPA in Fig. 5.1)**.

Fixation Axis

This is a straight line that joins center of rotation of eyeball with fixation point **(VC in Fig. 5.1)**.

Angles (Fig. 5.1)

- Angle Alpha is the angle formed between optical axis and visual axis, i.e., angle ONV.
- Angle Kappa is the angle formed between visual axis and pupillary axis.
- Angle Gamma is the angle formed between optical axis and fixation axis, i.e., angle OCV.

Purkinje Images (Catoptric Imagery)

These were first described by a Czech scientist JE Purkinje to differentiate between aphakia and normal eye. These are four in number and are formed as a result of reflection from different ocular surfaces **(Fig. 5.2)**.

First Purkinje image	Formed by reflection from anterior surface of cornea, situated near pupillary plane. It is brightest, virtual and erect image. This image is made use of in keratometry
Second Purkinje image	Formed by reflection from posterior surface of cornea, situated near pupillary plane. It is virtual and erect image
Third Purkinje image	Formed by reflection from anterior surface of lens, situated in vitreous. It is the largest but dim, virtual and erect image
Fourth Purkinje image	Formed by reflection from posterior surface of lens, situated within the lens. It is real and inverted image. It moves in opposite direction to other images

Clinical Applications

- To diagnose presence or absence of lens.
- Keratometry makes use of first Purkinje image.

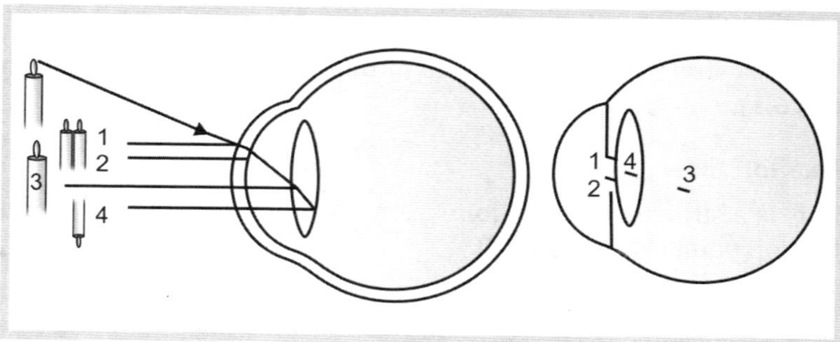

Fig. 5.2: Purkinje images.

- **Type of cataract:** In MSC and HMSC, Fourth Purkinje image is absent.
- **Hirschberg test:** First Purkinje image is used for estimation of angle of squint.

6 CHAPTER

Refractive Errors

Parallel rays of light coming from infinity are focused on retina under normal conditions and thus the image of an object is formed on retina. This condition is known as emmetropia. This image is very small in size and inverted. From retina, this image is carried to brain via optic nerve where it is re-inverted and interpreted by visual cortex. Vision of person is recorded as 6/6 on Snellen's chart and the power of eyeball is +60 Diopter. If parallel rays of light coming from infinity are not focused on retina; the condition is known as ametropia or a state of refractive error. Different types of refractive errors are shown in **Figure 6.1**:

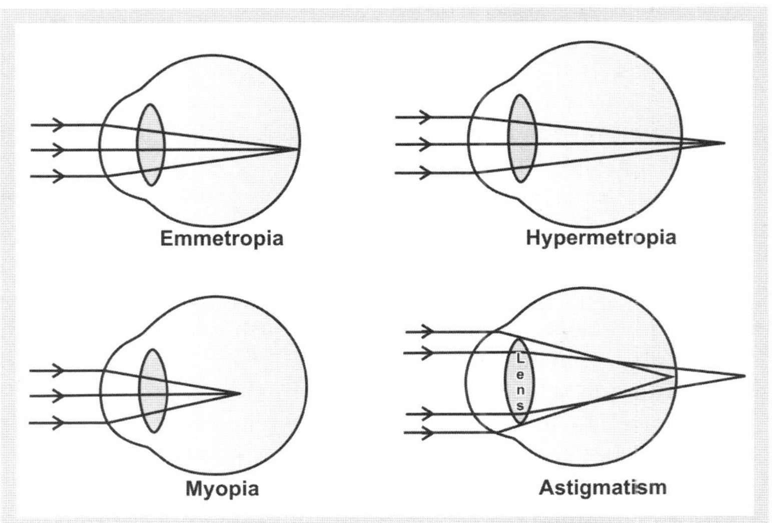

Fig. 6.1: Different types of refractive errors.

- Myopia
- Hypermetropia
- Astigmatism

MYOPIA

This is also known as 'Short Sightedness'. It is defined as a condition of refraction in which parallel rays of light coming from infinity are focused in front of retina with accommodation at rest. This is because the power of eyeball is more than +60D.

Types of Myopia

Depending upon mechanism of production, myopia may be of different types:

- **Axial myopia:** Here the axial length of eyeball is more than normal (>24 mm). One mm increase in axial length causes three diopter of myopia.
- **Curvature myopia:** Curvature of cornea or lens is more than normal. One mm increase in curvature causes six diopter of myopia. Keratoconus and lenticonus are clinical entities which cause high curvature myopia.
- **Index myopia:** Refractive index of eyeball is more than normal, e.g., in nuclear sclerosis refractive index of lens is increased causing a myopic shift.
- **Positional myopia:** Anterior displacement of lens in the eyeball causes a myopic shift.
- Excessive accommodation as occurs in spasm of accommodation causes myopia.

Depending upon clinical presentation myopia may be of different types:

- **Congenital myopia:** It is present since birth but parents come to know about the disease at around 2 to 3 years of age. The child usually requires high concave lens (8–10D) to correct the error. It may be unilateral or bilateral. The child may develop convergent squint. It may also be associated with other congenital anomalies like microphthalmos, microcornea, congenital cataract etc.
- **Simple myopia:** This is the most common variety of myopia encountered clinically. Patients may complain of blurring of vision, eyestrain while reading, writing or working on computer

and watching television. The school going child may complain of doing mistakes when he copies matter written on black board. If error is small, eyestrain symptoms occur more because he tries to compensate for the error and if error is of high degree, patient is not able to see distant objects. On examination, myopic eyeball is more prominent with large pupils. Fundus may show temporal crescent. Diagnosis is confirmed by retinoscopy.

- **Pathological myopia:** This is also known as degenerative myopia. There is rapid progress of myopia in early adult life associated with degenerative changes of retina and vitreous. It occurs due to rapid increase in axial length of eyeball. Heredity plays the main role because this type of myopia is more common in persons with family history of high myopia. It is more common in some races like Japanese, Chinese and it is less common in Negroes and Sudanese. Due to rapid growth sclera follows the growth of retina but choroid undergoes degeneration followed by degeneration of retina.

  General factors like nutritional deficiency, debilitating diseases, wrong posture, poor illumination, and working on computer for long hours play a minor role in progress of myopia.

Symptoms and Signs of Degenerative Myopia

- A patient of progressive myopia complains of rapid deterioration of vision, vision may not improve to normal status.
- Muscae volitantes (a specific type of vitreous floater) and black opacities in front of eyes are complained of by many patients.
- Some patients may complain of night blindness due to degeneration of retina.
- Eyeball may appear proptosed in unilateral cases. Lengthening occurs mainly around posterior pole.
- Anterior chamber is deep and cornea may be bigger than normal.
- Pupils may be bigger in size and react sluggishly to light.
- Fundus may show big optic disk with temporal crescent **(Fig. 6.2)** or peripapillary atrophy. Retina becomes very thin and prone to rhegmatogenous retinal detachment. Foster-Fuch's spot (dark red spot due to subretinal neovascularization and choroidal hemorrhage) **(Fig. 6.4)** may be seen. Cystoid degeneration may occur in the peripheral retina. Posterior staphyloma **(Fig. 6.3)** may be formed due to ectasia of sclera at posterior pole lined by

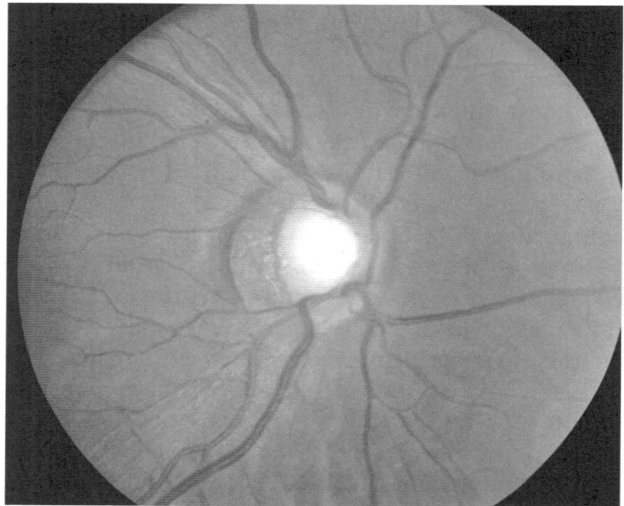

Fig. 6.2: Temporal crescent.

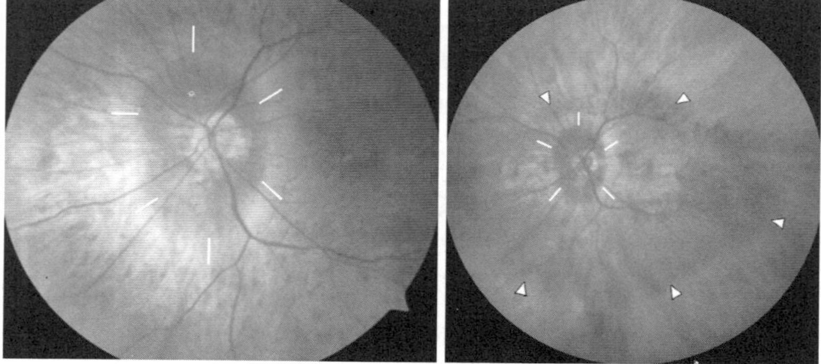

Fig. 6.3: Posterior staphyloma.

choroid and retina. In advanced cases retinal atrophy may occur and patient may go blind.

- Vitreous becomes liquefied with posterior vitreous detachment and vitreous opacities.
- Visual fields become contracted and ERG reveals subnormal reading due to chorioretinal degeneration.

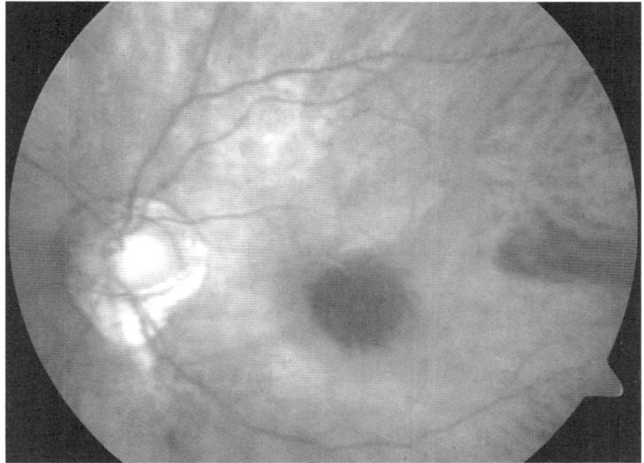

Fig. 6.4: Foster Fuch's spot.

Treatment of Myopia

Myopia is corrected by appropriate concave lenses either in form of spectacles or contact lens. Surgical correction of myopia can be done by photorefractive surgery or exchange of clear lens.

Contact lenses are cosmetically better suited with minimal aberrations and maximum visual field especially in high myopes. However they need motivation and better care on part of patient.

LASIK laser surgery is gaining popularity day by day. But it has its own limitations, as very high myopes are sometimes not fit for surgery due to poor corneal thickness or keratoconus.

Very high myopia can be rectified by *lens exchange* but patient has to accept bifocal lenses in young age because accommodation is lost after surgery.

Recent development in treatment of very high myopia is *implantable contact lens*. In this surgery normal lens is left as such and through a limbal incision an implantable contact lens is fitted over the normal crystalline lens. This contact lens keeps on floating over the crystalline lens. It is an alternative to LASIK laser surgery where thickness of cornea is a limiting factor. Thus patient gets rid of spectacles and accommodation is also retained. However this surgery is quite costly.

Recently special types of contact lenses have been introduced called the *ortho-k* lenses which are to be used by the patient overnight and removed during day time. This corrects myopia as well as hypermetropia in a reversible manner. Once the patient stops using them the refractive error returns back.

Combination of clear lens extraction and LASIK laser can also be done in very high myopes. However accommodation is lost.

Thus every patient should be individualized for type of treatment.

While correcting myopia the basic rule must be followed everywhere that myopia is always under corrected to avoid minification and reading difficulties.

Low vision aids are prescribed to patients who cannot carry out their routine activities even with glasses. These are special types of spectacles, which are prescribed to patients with very poor vision.

Prevention of progressive myopia can be done at community level by marriage counseling. A progressive myope should not marry another progressive myope or they should not bear children.

Myopia control measures: A lot of research is going on Myopia Control. Some of them are described below:

- **Low dose atropine** eye drops (0.01%) have been advocated to slow down progress of myopia and are freely available in Indian market. It is used at night in children between 5 to 18 years of age. Exact mechanism of action is not known but it is supposed to slow down elongation of eyeball which in turn retards progress of axial myopia. Low dose atropine slightly dilates the pupil so that there is no photophobia and no remarkable loss of accommodation. It alters the peripheral defocus pattern of retina. When a child is born the size of eyeball is very small and rays of light are focused behind the retina, means the child is hypermetropic. This is known as **hyperopic defocus**. This hyperopic defocus is a trigger for axial lengthening of eyeball. Even in an emmetropic eyeball where rays of light are focused on retina, the peripheral rays are still focused behind the retina because the vertical height of eyeball is lesser than axial length of eyeball. This is known as **peripheral hyperopic defocus** which again is a trigger for axial lengthening of eyeball. Low dose atropine alters peripheral hyperopic defocus patterns and helps retard lengthening of eyeball. Further research is still going on exact concentration and dose of atropine and age of patient for optimum results. Research is also being done on Pirenzepine gel for its role in myopia control.

- **Myopia control lenses (Fig. 6.5):** These lenses are being manufactured by Hoya, Essilor, Cooper Vision, and Zeiss. These lenses are based on the principle of creating peripheral myopic defocus which slows down the axial lengthening of eyeball. The lens consists of exact prescription as per refractive error of the patient in its central part so that this part creates emmetropia. It is meant to see central field of vision. This part is surrounded by rings of small highly aspherical lenslets. These lenslets are designed in such a way that they have lesser power as compared to the prescription of the patient. Thus, these lenslets make the rays of light focus in front of retina. Again, there is a space between two rings of lenslets which creates emmetropia so that there is no constriction of visual field. In a nutshell 60% of the total area of lens creates emmetropia and 40% creates myopic defocus. When rays of light are focused in front of retina, it sends a signal to the brain that there is no need of further elongation of eyeball and thus progress of myopia is slowed down. However, research is still going on to exactly understand its mechanism of action. **Progressive addition lenses** are also prescribed to children for

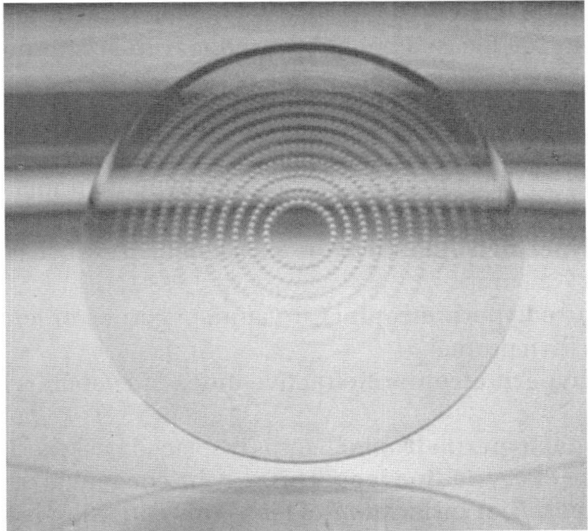

Fig. 6.5: Myopia control lens.

control of myopia. This is again based on same principle of altering peripheral defocus.

- **Orthokeratology:** Ortho K lenses when given to patient at night flatten the central part of cornea and alter peripheral hyperopic defocus pattern due to its mechanical pressure and some biochemical changes produced in the corneal tissue. This reduces the dependence of patient on spectacles.
- **Modification of lifestyle:** This is again very important aspect of myopia control. A surge in myopia has been noticed in post covid era. It has been suggested that working on digital gadgets like mobile, laptop, etc., indoor activities, reading or writing in lying down position, low illumination put strain on eyeball and add to lengthening of eyeball. Hence, it is suggested that every child should be encouraged to play outside in natural light at least for two hours a day in addition to his school hours.

Complications of Pathological Myopia

These are retinal detachment, vitreous degeneration, and complicated cataract.

HYPERMETROPIA

This is a type of refractive error in which parallel rays of light coming from infinity are focused behind the retina with accommodation at rest. Power of eyeball is less than normal (< +60D).

Types of Hypermetropia

Depending on mechanism of production, hypermetropia can be of different types:

- **Axial hypermetropia:** Here the axial length of eyeball is less than normal (<24 mm).
- **Curvature hypermetropia:** Curvature of cornea or lens or both are less than normal.
- **Index hypermetropia:** Refractive index of eyeball is less than normal.
- **Positional hypermetropia:** Lens is displaced backwards.
- **Absence of crystalline lens:** This may be congenital or acquired due to posterior dislocation of lens. This condition is known as aphakia.

Depending on clinical presentation hypermetropia can be of different types:

- **Simple hypermetropia:** This is due to normal biological variation in development of eyeball. This is the most common type of hypermetropia.
- **Pathological hypermetropia:** This is due to certain factors which are not in the normal biological variations, e.g., posterior subluxation of lens (positional hypermetropia), acquired cortical sclerosis (index hypermetropia), under-correction of refractive error (consecutive hypermetropia) and congenital absence of lens (aphakia).
- **Functional hypermetropia:** It results due to paralysis of accommodation, e.g., third nerve paralysis.

Components of Hypermetropia

Total Hypermetropia

Total amount of hypermetropia estimated after complete cycloplegia with atropine. It has two parts latent and manifest.

Latent Hypermetropia

This part is corrected by inherent ciliary tone. It is usually one diopter. It is more in children and decreases with age.

Manifest

This part of hypermetropia cannot be corrected by ciliary tone. It has two components.

1. **Facultative:** This part of hypermetropia can be corrected by accommodative effort.
2. **Absolute:** This part of hypermetropia cannot be corrected by accommodative effort.

Example

Suppose a patient is put atropine eye ointment and full cycloplegia is achieved. Now retinoscopy findings at one meter distance show +6.00 DS in both horizontal and vertical meridia. So total hypermetropia in this patient will be +6–1(distance factor) = +5 DS +1.00 DS is the latent hypermetropia due to inherent ciliary tone and manifest hypermetropia is +5–1= +4.00 DS. Now if patient accepts +2.50 DS with 6/6 vision (best corrected vision), then +2.50 DS is the absolute hypermetropia which cannot be corrected by accommodative effort and patient needs glasses.

+4.00–2.50 = +1.50 DS is the facultative hypermetropia which patient corrected with his accommodative effort (minimum power of convex lens required to achieve best vision is absolute hypermetropia and maximum power of convex lens required to achieve best vision is manifest hypermetropia. Manifest – Absolute = Facultative hypermetropia).

Clinical Features of Hypermetropia

Symptoms depend on the amount of hypermetropia and age of person. These may be:

- **Asymptomatic:** A person who does not have much visual requirement and has a small refractive error may not complain of any problem and refractive error may be detected just by chance.
- **Eyestrain:** Patient complains of headache, watering, tiredness of eyes while working on computer, watching television and doing reading and writing work. This is due to sustained accommodative effort.
- **Defective vision:** When amount of error is very high; patient may not try to compensate it and complains of defective vision. If patient can compensate some amount of error by accommodative effort and rest of the error remains uncompensated; he may complain of eyestrain symptoms and defective vision both more for near than for distance.
- On examination size of eyeball appears smaller with small cornea, shallow anterior chamber and small optic disk with indistinct margins (pseudopapillitis). Retina shows more shining called 'Shot-Silk Retina'. Axial length can be confirmed with A-Scan.

Management of Hypermetropia

Diagnosis is confirmed by retinoscopy under cycloplegia. Fogging test should be done and maximum acceptance should be prescribed. However, patient should be comfortable with the prescription. Cylinder should be prescribed fully. If patient is not comfortable with full correction at first sitting; under correction may be done with small increment after a gap of three to six months. Full correction must be given at first sitting if patient is having accommodative squint.

This error is corrected by prescribing convex lens so that the rays are converged and focused on retina. Convex lens can be prescribed in form of *spectacles, contact lens, refractive corneal surgery, phakic IOLs and ortho-k lenses.*

Phakic IOL is a type of IOL which is implanted over and above the normal transparent crystalline lens. However, the surgery is a bit tricky and should be done by expert hand as it can damage the normal lens and make it cataractous. This procedure is done to correct very high hypermetropia.

ASTIGMATISM

It is a type of refractive error in which parallel rays of light coming from infinity do not come to a focus but form focal lines with accommodation at rest. This is because the refractive power is different in different meridia.

Types of Astigmatism

Astigmatism is of two types **(Flowchart 6.1)**:

1. **Regular astigmatism:** Refractive power changes uniformly from one meridian to another. It has two principal meridia. It can be corrected by spectacles, contact lens and refractive surgery.
2. **Irregular astigmatism:** Refractive power does not change uniformly from one meridian to another. It cannot be corrected by spectacles and semisoft contact lenses should be advised.

Flowchart 6.1: Types of astigmatism.

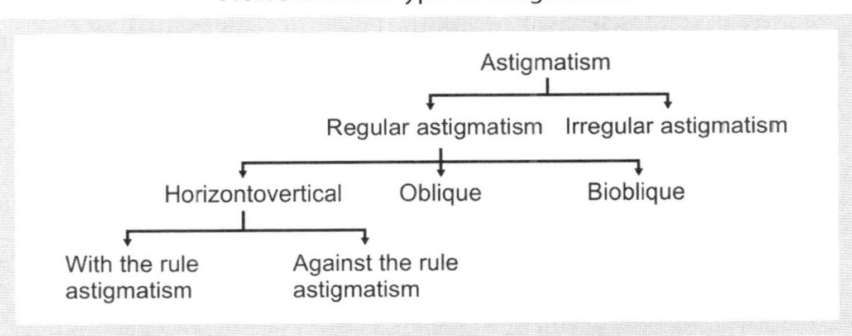

Types of Regular Astigmatism

- **Horizontovertical:** Here the two principal meridia are horizontal and vertical. If the vertical meridian is more curved (hence more power) than horizontal meridian, it is called 'with the rule' astigmatism. This is called 'with the rule' because vertical meridian is generally more curved due to pressure of lids on eyeball. This type of astigmatism is corrected by minus cylinder at 180° or plus cylinder at 90°. If horizontal meridian is more curved than vertical meridian, it is called 'against the rule' astigmatism. This type of astigmatism is corrected by minus cylinder at 90° or plus cylinder at 180°.
- **Oblique astigmatism:** Here the two principal meridia are not horizontal or vertical but still they are placed at right angle to each other, e.g., the two meridia can be 45° and 135° or 10° and 100°.
- **Bioblique astigmatism:** Here the two principal meridia are oblique and at the same time, they do not intersect at right angle to each other, e.g., one meridian may be at 10° and other at 30°. This type of astigmatism cannot be corrected by spectacles.

Depending upon at which point the rays of light are focused, astigmatism can be of different types (Fig. 6.6):

- **Simple myopic astigmatism:** One meridian is focused on retina and the other is focused in front of retina, e.g,. –1.00 DC at 180° prescription shows that it is a case of simple myopic astigmatism.
- **Simple hypermetropic astigmatism:** One meridian is focused at retina and the other is focused behind the retina, e.g., +1.00 DC at 180° prescription shows that it is a case of simple hypermetropic astigmatism.
- **Compound myopic astigmatism:** Both the principal meridia are focused in front of retina, e.g., –1.00DS/–1.00DC at 180° prescription shows that it is a case of compound myopic astigmatism.
- **Compound hypermetropic astigmatism:** Both the principal meridia are focused behind the retina, e.g., +1.00DS/+1.00DC at 180° prescription shows that it is a case of compound hypermetropic astigmatism.
- **Mixed astigmatism:** One meridian is focused in front of retina and the other is focused behind the retina, e.g., +1.00DS/–2.00DC at 180° prescription shows that, it is a case of mixed astigmatism.

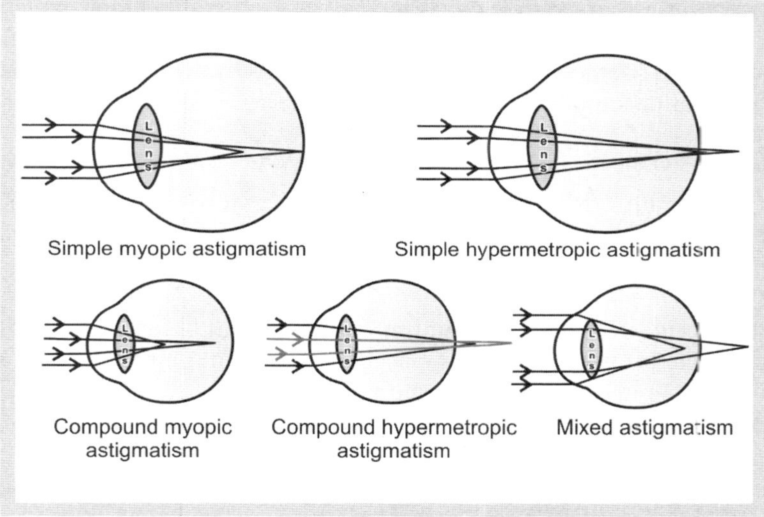

Fig. 6.6: Types of astigmatism.

Depending upon etiology, astigmatism can be:

- **Corneal astigmatism:** Abnormality lies in the anatomy of cornea.
- **Lenticular astigmatism:** It may occur due to tilting of lens or abnormal curvature of lens (lenticonus).
- **Retinal astigmatism:** Due to oblique placement of macula as may occur in scarring of retina.

Clinical Features

- Patient may complain of eyeache, headache, tiredness of eyes and sometimes nausea if the error is small. These are known as asthenopic symptoms.
- Blurring of vision and distorted appearance of objects may be complained of by some persons.

Treatment

Astigmatism can be corrected either by glasses or by contact lens or corneal refractive surgery. Regular astigmatism can be corrected by spectacles. However if the cylindrical power is high (2-3D) the quality of vision is better with semisoft contact lens as compared to glasses. For very high astigmatism Toric contact lens can be prescribed.

Irregular astigmatism is corrected by semisoft contact lens, which replaces the irregular anterior surface of cornea with regular surface of contact lens. If vision does not improve with contact lens penetrating keratoplasty should be considered.

Strum's Conoid

Configuration of rays when they get refracted through a sphero-cylindrical surface (toric or compound lens) is like the shape of a cone hence called the Strum's conoid. It has the following features **(Fig. 6.7)**:

- A toric surface has maximum curvature and hence maximum power in one meridian (suppose vertical) and minimum curvature in other meridian (suppose horizontal).
- When parallel rays of light pass through a convex toric lens, vertical rays get focused at point M and horizontal rays get focused at point N. Thus these rays have two foci. The distance between the two foci is called 'Focal interval of strum.'
- If these rays are intercepted at different points A, B, C, D, E, and F, a circular object will appear as shown in the **Figure 6.7**.

Now if retina is presumed to be present at point A, the condition becomes compound hypermetropic astigmatism where both the meridia are getting focused behind the retina.

If retina is at point B, it is simple hypermetropic astigmatism where vertical rays have come to a focus but horizontal rays are yet to focus.

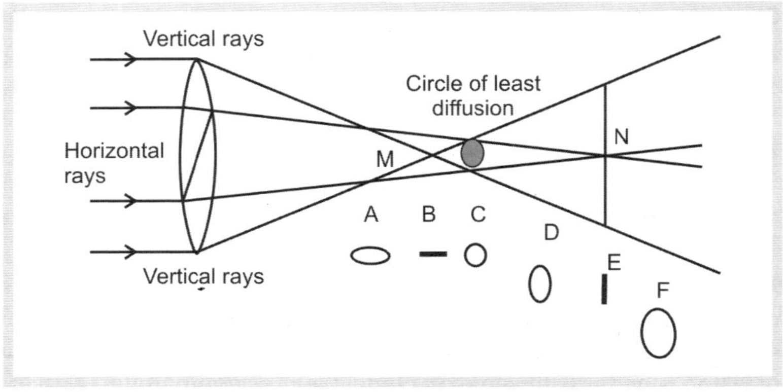

Fig. 6.7: Strum's conoid.

If retina is at point C, it is a condition of mixed astigmatism where vertical rays have focused in front of retina and horizontal rays get focused behind the retina.

If retina is at point E, it is simple myopic astigmatism, where vertical rays have focused in front of retina and horizontal rays have focused on retina.

If retina is at point F, it becomes a case of compound myopic astigmatism where both the meridia have focused in front of retina.

Clinical Significance

It explains why an astigmatic patient complains of seeing distorted objects. Also that a patient having mixed astigmatism may not complain of defective vision as the circle of least diffusion falls on his retina and hence his visual acuity is very good even without glasses.

APHAKIA

It is absence of crystalline lens in its normal position in the eyeball. It may be congenital absence of crystalline lens or acquired (surgical removal of lens as after cataract surgery). It creates a high degree of hypermetropia.

Causes

- Congenital absence of crystalline lens.
- Surgical aphakia, e.g., after cataract surgery.
- **Traumatic aphakia:** Lens is expelled out due to some injury.
- Spontaneous absorption of lens may occur sometimes producing aphakia.
- Posterior dislocation of lens in the vitreous cavity.

Clinical Features

Patient complains of marked loss of vision for distance and near, as there is total loss of accommodation. On examination:

- Surgical scar mark may be seen on limbus.
- Anterior chamber is deep.
- Iris shows tremulousness (iridodonesis) on movement of eyeball.
- Pupil is jet black in color.

- 3rd and 4th Purkinje images are absent.
- Fundus shows small disk with indistinct disk margins.
- Retinoscopy shows high hypermetropia.

Treatment

It can be corrected by glasses, contact lens and intraocular lens implantation. Usually +10 DS lens along with cylinder for induced astigmatism is required to correct aphakia in a previously emmetropic patient. However, each and every patient should be individually assessed by retinoscopy for the power of glasses required. Aphakic glasses have the advantage of being cheap, safe and easy method of rehabilitation of aphakia. However there are a lot of problems associated with use of these glasses. These are magnification of image by 30% thus totally unfit for unilateral aphakia as this causes diplopia. It also causes hand eye incoordination, problems of spherical and chromatic aberration due to thickness of lens. Field of vision is limited. There is prismatic effect from edges of glass. Objects appear and disappear if the patient tries to see them by moving eyes, i.e., roving ring scotoma (jack in box phenomenon). So patient should be advised to move his head instead of moving his eyes to look sideways. Cosmetically they are unacceptable especially in young persons.

Somewhat better method is use of *contact lenses*. They are cosmetically acceptable with less magnification (7%), more suited for unilateral aphakia with wider and better field of vision. Spherical and chromatic aberrations are absent. However they are costly, difficult to wear especially for old bilateral aphakes. Very good personal hygiene is required.

The best method of rehabilitation of aphakia is *IOL implantation.* It is fitted on the table during surgery. It can also be implanted later on as secondary IOL implantation. It has 1 to 2% magnification only, hardly appreciated by patient, no aberration, no prismatic effect. That is why they are becoming more and more popular. However special training needs to be given to the surgeon for good results and costly equipments are required for surgery.

Another method of rehabilitation of aphakia is refractive corneal surgery. LASIK laser is the best modality. In this surgery corneal stroma is ablated with laser to alter its curvature and thus alter the power of eyeball. Keratophakia and epikeratophakia have still not gained popularity.

PSEUDOPHAKIA

It is a condition of eyeball when an artificial lens is present in place of crystalline lens.

Types of IOLs

Depending upon position of IOL they are of different types **(Fig. 6.8)**:

- **AC-IOL (anterior chamber):** It may be angle supported or iris supported IOL, e.g., Iris claw lens.
- **PC-IOL (posterior chamber):** It may be 'in-the-bag' IOL, Sulcus (between iris and anterior capsule of lens) fixated IOL or Scleral fixated IOL **(Fig. 6.9)**.
  'In-the-bag' IOL is the best IOL because it is the natural position of lens.

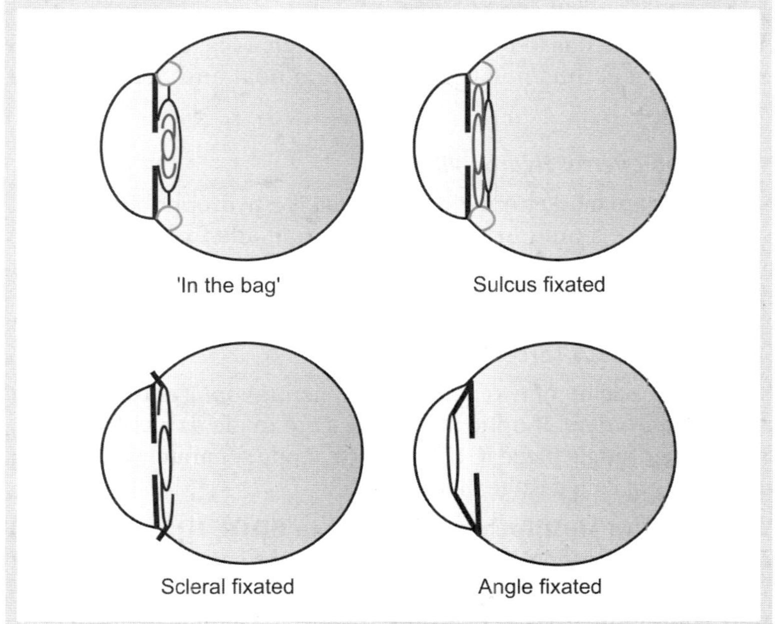

Fig. 6.8: Types of IOLs.

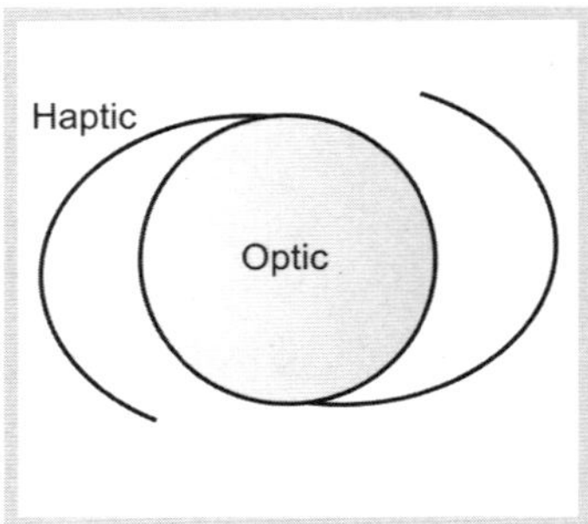

Fig. 6.9: Design of PC-IOL.

Foldable versus Nonfoldable IOL

Foldable IOLs are made from silicone and acrylic and can be folded without changing its optical properties. Such types of IOLs can be injected through a very small hole on limbus (2.8 mm or even less). Inside the posterior chamber they unfold and can be implanted in the bag. Nonfoldable IOL is made from Poly (methyl methacrylate) (PMMA) and needs to be implanted through a bigger incision (5.25 mm or bigger) thus needs more time to heal and there is more astigmatism.

Hydrophobic versus Hydrophilic IOLs

Some IOLs are made from PMMA, which is a hydrophobic material. Such IOLs are stored dry. Other IOLs are made from hydrophilic material and stored in solution. There are less chances of after cataract with hydrophobic material.

Single Piece versus Three Piece IOL

An IOL is made up of two parts namely central *optic* and peripheral parts called *haptic*. If optic and haptics are made as a single piece, this is called single piece IOL. If they are made separately and joined later, they are called three piece IOL.

Monofocal vs Multifocal vs Trifocal vs EDOF IOLs (Figs. 6.10 and 6.11): Monofocal IOLs are meant to take care of either distant or near vision and patient needs glasses after surgery. This is the most commonly used IOL as on today because they are less costly and there is no issue of glare at night. The whole IOL contains only

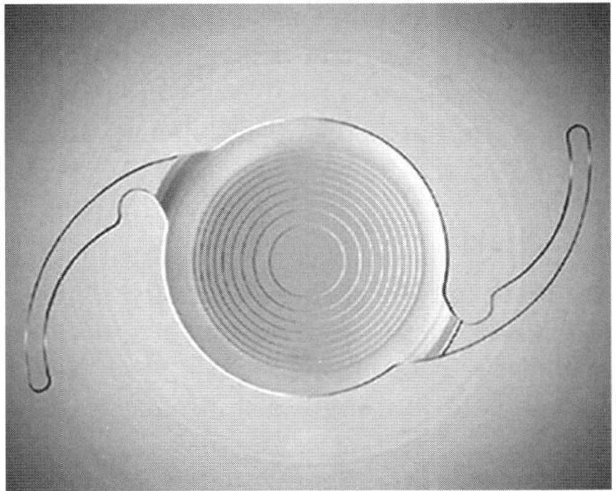

Fig. 6.10: Multifocal IOL.

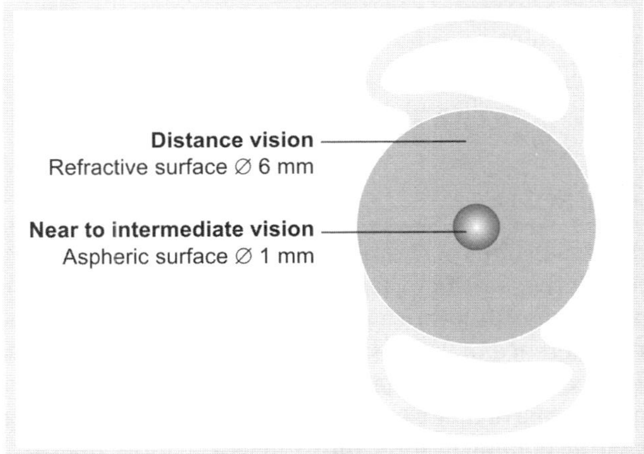

Fig. 6.11: EDOFF IOL with a central hump.

one power on its surface. **In Multifocal/Bifocal IOLs** both distant and near vision are corrected and there is minimal dependence on glasses after surgery. **In Trifocal IOLs**, distant, intermediate and near vision, all are corrected by the IOL. It is required by patients who use digital gadgets in their routine activities. Multifocal and trifocal designs are created by refractive and diffractive rings visible on the IOL surface. However multifocal and trifocal IOLs are not advised to persons who drive at night because they create glare. **Extended depth of focus (EDOF)** IOLs are created either by inducing spherical aberration in the central part of IOL or by creating a hump in the central one mm of the IOL. This design has an advantage of glare free vision even at night.

Signs of Pseudophakia

- Surgical scar mark may be visible on limbus.
- AC appears slightly deeper than normal.
- Mild iridodonesis may be appreciated.
- Pupil is black in color but it gives shining reflex when examined with torchlight.
- Visual status depends on refractive status achieved after surgery.
- Slit-lamp examination with dilated pupil confirms the diagnosis.

Residual Error

Usually, a patient has some spherical and cylindrical error left after IOL implantation even in the best of hands. Spherical error can be removed by accurate biometry and cylindrical error can be minimized by decreasing the size of incision.

ANISOMETROPIA

When refractive status of two eyes is equal, it is known as isometropia. When refractive status of two eyes is not equal, it is known as anisometropia. A difference of 1D in refractive status of two eyes creates a difference of 2% in size of retinal image of two eyes. Up to 5% difference in retinal image size of two eyes is well tolerated. Thus an anisometropia of up to 2.5D is acceptable. Anisometropia of up to 4D may be acceptable in some individuals and more than 4D creates diplopia.

Causes

It may be congenital or developmental or acquired as in unilateral aphakia.

Clinical Significance

Small degree of anisometropia is of no concern and is quite common. Patient develops normal binocular single vision. However, if one eye is emmetropic and other is highly hypermetropic, the later will develop suppression and amblyopia (lazy eye). Patient will use only emmetropic eye for vision. If one eye is myopic and other is hypermetropic, then patient will develop alternate vision. It means that he will use myopic eye for near vision and hypermetropic eye for distant vision.

Types of Anisometropia

- **Simple anisometropia:** Here one eye is normal (vision 6/6 without glasses) and other eye is myopic, e.g., 6/6 vision with -2.00DS. It is known as simple myopic anisometropia. If other eye is hypermetropic e.g., 6/6 vision with +2.00DS, it is known as simple hypermetropic anisometropia.
- **Compound anisometropia:** Here both eyes are either myopic (compound myopic anisometropia; one eye requires -2.00DS and other -5.00DS) or hypermetropic (compound hypermetropic anisometropia; one eye requires +2.00DS and other –5.00DS) but one eye has higher refractive error than the other.
- **Mixed anisometropia:** Here one eye is myopic and other eye is hypermetropic, e.g., one eye requires -2.00DS and other eye requires +2.00DS.

Diagnosis and Treatment of Anisometropia

Patient is diagnosed on retinoscopy. He may complain of defective vision, headache and other eyestrain symptoms. Different types of treatment modalities available are:

Spectacles

Care should be taken that patient does not have diplopia or eyestrain while prescribing glasses. A difference of up to 4D can be tolerated.

Contact Lens

Higher degree of anisometropia can be corrected by contact lenses.

Others

Refractive corneal surgery can be done, IOL can be implanted if there is unilateral aphakia, and exchange of crystalline lens can be done if there is high hypermetropia or high myopia. Phakic IOL can be done in very high hypermetropia. Two procedures can also be combined if required.

ANISEIKONIA

It is a condition when images projected on visual cortex from two eyes are unequal in size or shape. Up to 5% aniseikonia can be well tolerated.

Types (Figs. 6.12 and 6.13)

It may be *optical aniseikonia* when image size difference is due to anisometropia, *retinal aniseikonia* due to displacement of retinal elements towards nodal point as a result of retinal edema and *cortical aniseikonia* due to abnormality in perception of image. Causes of retinal aniseikonia are macular pucker, central serous retinopathy, RD repair, epiretinal membrane, solar burn and macular degeneration.

It can be further of two types: **symmetrical** when one image is larger than the other in all dimensions **(spherical aniseikonia)** or in one dimension **(cylindrical aniseikonia)**, e.g., if one eye sees a square the other eye may see the square with bigger length and breadth or only length may be larger. In **asymmetrical** aniseikonia image may be distorted in some degree, it may be progressively larger in one

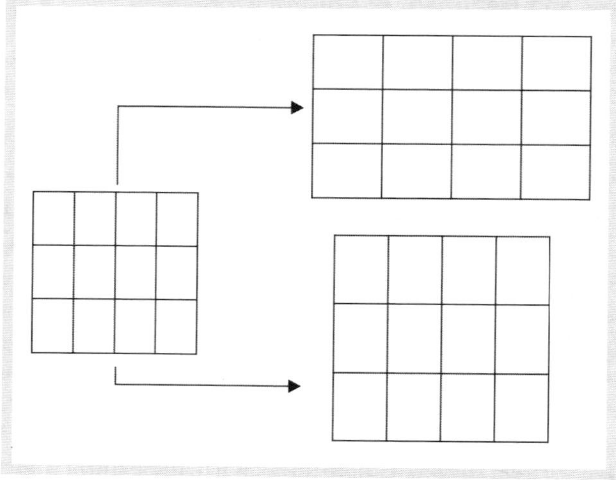

Fig. 6.12: Symmetrical aniseikonia.

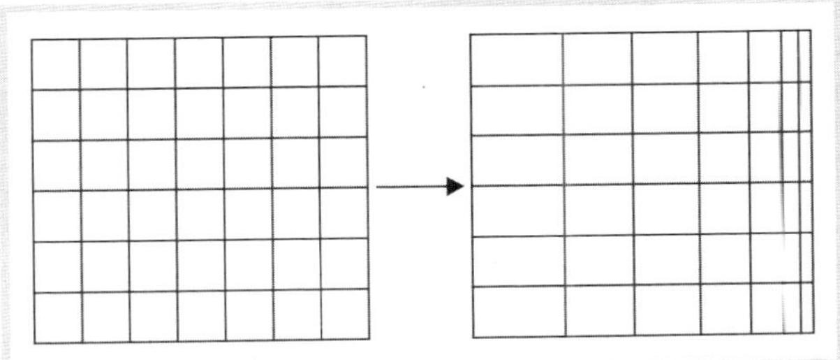

Fig. 6.13: Asymmetrical aniseikonia.

dimension and smaller in other dimension. Asymmetrical aniseikonia can be **prismatic type:** Image size increases progressively in one direction, **Pincushion distortion type:** As occurs with Aphakic glasses, **barrel-shaped distortion type:** As occurs with high minus lenses and **oblique:** Size of image is same but there is oblique distortion.

Clinical features: These are eyestrain symptoms like problems in reading, writing, working on mobile, computer, etc., headache, photophobia, dizziness, nausea, disorientation, nervousness, physical fatigue and inability to see 3D images, diplopia, confusion and vertigo if the difference in image size is more than 5% and there is difficulty in depth perception. Aniseikonia can be measured by space eikonometer but it is not popular as the method is costly, cumbersome and of little therapeutic value. Clinically, it is measured by a thumb rule that 1Diopter of anisometropia creates 2% of aniseikonia.

Treatment

Optical aniseikonia can be treated by contact lens, IOL implantation and corneal refractive surgery. Aniseikonic spectacles which cause magnification of image without introducing any appreciable power are also a method of treatment. Retinal aniseikonia needs treatment of cause. Cortical aniseikonia is very difficult to treat.

Aniseikonic glasses also known as size lenses, which magnify image without introducing appreciable power. They are made by changing parameters like base curve, central thickness and vertex distance. They are best suited for isometric aniseikonia, which means when axial length is the primary cause of aniseikonia. If change in keratometry reading is the primary cause of aniseikonia, contact lenses are the best method to treat aniseikonia.

AMBLYOPIA OR LAZY EYE

It is a type of functional abnormality of visual system in which one or both eyeballs are affected. Vision does not improve beyond a certain limit and no physical abnormality of ocular media or visual pathway can be blamed for poor vision. About 1–4% of children suffer from this abnormality.

Types of Amblyopia

It is of different types:

- **Stimulus deprivation amblyopia:** If a child has congenital cataract, corneal opacity or any other opacity in the media so that the rays of light do not pass and focus on retina, the child will develop amblyopia. This is because the retina has been deprived of the light stimulus in early childhood that is very much essential for normal functioning of retina. This type of amblyopia is least common but most difficult to treat. It has been seen in experiments on animals that there is shrinkage of cells of lateral geniculate body and visual cortex in response to amblyopia hence most difficult to treat. Again, unilateral amblyopia is more difficult to treat than bilateral amblyopia because in bilateral amblyopia there is no abnormal binocular interaction (due to disparity of images of two eyes) but only form vision and light deprivation that needs to be treated. Light deprivation, form vision deprivation and abnormal binocular interaction are also known as amblyogenic factors.
- **Strabismic amblyopia:** If a child has squint or strabismus, one eye dominates over the other causing suppression, which consequently becomes amblyopic. It is more common in esotropia than exotropia. It is because the temporal retina (fovea) has more cone density and has better vision as compared to nasal retina. In esotropia, image that falls on fovea of normal eye also falls on nasal retina of squinting eye. Thus, weak nasal retina of squinting eye has to compete with stronger fovea of normal eye. In case of exotropia, an image that falls on fovea of squinting eye, also falls on weaker nasal retina of normal eye thus a stronger fovea of squinting eye needs to compete with weaker nasal retina of normal eye. It never occurs in alternate strabismus. Grating acuity is better than Snellen's acuity as recognizing presence of grating is a much simpler task than recognizing whole letter. Because cones become less sensitive in amblyopia and rods try to take over function of cones hence patient reads better with neutral density filter with amblyopic eye as compared to normal eye.

- **Anisometropic amblyopia:** If a child has anisometropia, i.e., one eye is emmetropic and another eye is high hypermetropic as in unilateral aphakia. It is suggested that there is form vision deprivation and abnormal binocular interaction caused by unequal images of two eyes that leads to this type of amblyopia.
- **B/L ametropic amblyopia:** If there is hypermetropia more than +5D, myopia more than –10D and astigmatism more than 2.5D, patient does not read 6/6 even with best correction. But if he uses glasses regularly, he is able to read 6/6 after some time without any kind of treatment. This is called bilateral ametropic amblyopia.
- **Meridional amblyopia:** This occurs in uncorrected astigmatic errors even if the error is of small degree.
- **Reverse amblyopia:** If normal eye is occluded for a long time in an effort to treat amblyopic eye early, the normal eye may also go into amblyopia. This is known as reverse amblyopia.

Diagnostic Criteria

- There must be a difference of two lines on Snellen's chart however any difference should be taken seriously.
- If a neutral density filter is placed before amblyopic eye, visual acuity improves in functional amblyopia but decreases in organic amblyopia. Loss of vision is reversible by occlusion therapy in functional amblyopia but not in organic amblyopia. However, these terms are no more used.
- Crowding phenomenon: If letters are crowded together, amblyopic eye finds it difficult to read.
- Color vision may be abnormal in severe amblyopia.

Risk factors for amblyopia: Children who have family history of amblyopia, premature birth or any other congenital abnormality are at a higher risk of developing amblyopia. Hence such patients should be thoroughly checked and followed up.

Treatment of Amblyopia

- **Correction of refractive error:** Correct the refractive error either by spectacles or contact lenses at the earliest possible.
- **Occlusion therapy:** Close the normal eye and patient is made to see with amblyopic eye. Duration of closure depends upon age of patient. It may be 5:1 or 4:1, i.e., normal eye is closed for five days and on sixth day amblyopic eye is closed so that the normal eye also gets chance to see and it may not become amblyopic. This occlusion is continued for minimum of three months or longer till the eye shows improvement.

- **Pleoptics:** It is a term introduced by Bangerter to include all types of treatment for amblyopia particularly that associated with eccentric fixation. This includes exercises like CAM stimulator and synoptophore exercises.
- A lot of research work is going on regarding treatment of amblyopia. Certain exercises on **Orthoptec (Fig. 6.14)**, an equipment designed to aim at treating amblyopia at any age without occlusion therapy has been advocated by an Indian Ophthalmologist, Dr Santhan Gopal. It has given encouraging results. It not only treats amblyopia but also helps improve hand eye coordination and develop binocularity also. It is claimed to be beneficial even in the treatment of nystagmus also. However long-term studies need to be carried out to evaluate its efficacy in the treatment of different conditions. Similarly **virtual realty (VR)** has emerged as a promising tool in the treatment of amblyopia. Because it is in form of games on digital screen, it is very easy to keep the child engaged. Different studies published in Journal of American Medical Association Ophthalmology in 2016, Investigative Ophthalmology & Visual Science in 2019 and Journal of Binocular Vision and Ocular Motility in 2020 endorse the usefulness of this treatment.

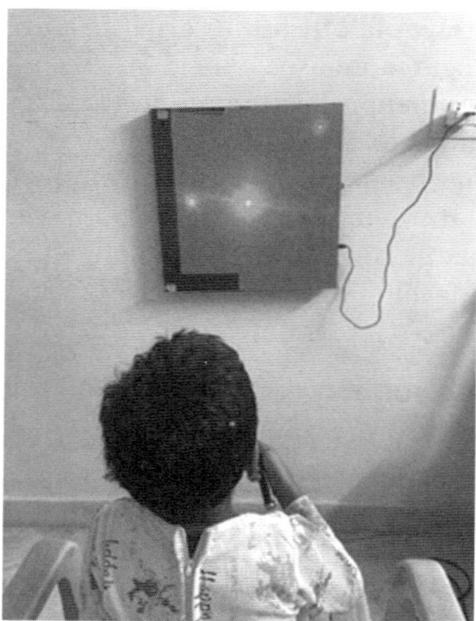

Fig. 6.14: Orthoptec.

Conventional treatment of amblyopia is possible before seven years of age. After that it becomes very difficult. Thus it is very important to detect amblyopia before this age. It is possible by a compulsory eye examination of child at the time of admission to school.

Why Myopia should be Slightly Under Corrected?

Myopia is corrected with a concave lens. A concave lens is a minifying lens. More is the power more is the minification caused by it. Thus myopia is always slightly under corrected to avoid minification of image and consequent eyestrain symptoms.

Why Hypermetropia should be Fully Corrected?

Hypermetropia should always be fully corrected so as to relax accommodation and avoid eyestrain symptoms. This is much more important in case of a squint. However it should be born in mind that correction is not done at the cost of producing eyestrain symptoms.

Near Objects Appear Clear to a Myopic Patient. Why?

This is because rays coming from a near object are divergent and more power is required to focus them on retina. As power of a myopic eyeball is >60D, hence rays are focused on retina and near objects appear clear to a myopic patient **(Fig. 6.15)**.

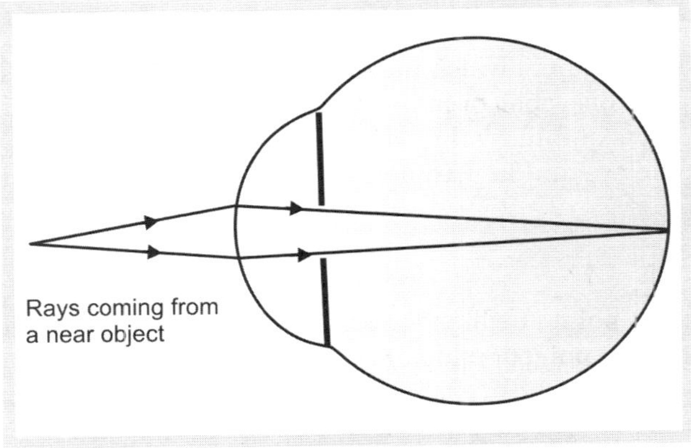

Fig. 6.15: Near vision and myopia.

Accommodation and Convergence

ACCOMMODATION

We know that parallel rays of light coming from a distant object are focused on our retina and we see distant objects clearly. At the same time when we look at a near object, again we can see it clearly. This is because our eyeball can increase or decrease its power. This inherent property of eyeball to increase or decrease its power is known as *accommodation*. This happens because when we see at a distant object our ciliary muscle is in a relaxed state, zonules are stretched apart and lens is less convex. Power of eyeball is +60D in an emmetropic eye. When we look at a near object our ciliary muscle contracts, zonules become loose and lens becomes more convex and thicker. Power of eyeball is increased to more than +60D. At rest radius of curvature of anterior and posterior surface of lens is 10 mm and 6 mm, respectively. When we accommodate it becomes 6 mm on both the surfaces.

Far Point

The farthest point at which the objects can be seen clearly is called the far point of eyeball or punctum remotum. In an emmetropic eye far point lies at infinity, in hypermetropic eye it is virtual and lies behind the eye and in myopic eye it is real and lies in front of the eyeball.

Near Point

The nearest point at which the small objects can be seen clearly is called the near point or punctum proximum. In emmetropic eye near point lies close to the eyeball depending on age. At 10 years of age, it is 7 cm, and at 40 years of age, it is 25 cm. Since we keep the reading material at 25 cm distance hence we can read without any aid till forty years of age. After that the near point recedes back and in order to read it clearly at 25 cm we need plus lenses. This condition of failing accommodation that occurs with increasing age is called presbyopia. This happens because the lens becomes less elastic with age hence cannot change its curvature and weakness of ciliary muscle. Certain conditions like open angle glaucoma, uncorrected hypermetropia can make the person presbyopic much earlier.

Range

The distance between the far point and the near point is called the range of accommodation.

Amplitude

Dioptric power of eyeball required to see at far point is lesser than the power required seeing at the near point. This difference in dioptric power of eyeball to see at near and distant object is known as amplitude of accommodation.

Mechanism

When we look at distant object our ciliary muscle is relaxed, distance between lens and ciliary muscle is more hence zonules are stretched. Curvature of anterior surface of lens is 10 mm and posterior surface is 6 mm. Power of eyeball in an emmetropic eye is +60 D. When we look at a near object ciliary muscle contracts, distance between lens and ciliary muscle is decreased hence zonules become lax, curvature of anterior and posterior surface of lens becomes 6 mm. Equatorial diameter of lens is decreased from 10 mm to 9.6 mm and thickness of lens is increased by 0.50 mm. Total power of eyeball is increased from 60 D to > +60 D. Lens is displaced slightly anteriorly by 0.30 mm hence AC becomes slightly shallow **(Figs. 7.1 and 7.2)**.

Facility of accommodation: It is how rapidly and accurately our eyes can respond to blur stimulus and make it clear. In other words, it is an adjustment that eye makes when it changes its fixation between distance and near target.

Theories of accommodation: Different theories of accommodation have been put forward to explain the mechanism of accommodation. According to **Helmholtz theory,** proposed by von Helmholtz in 19th

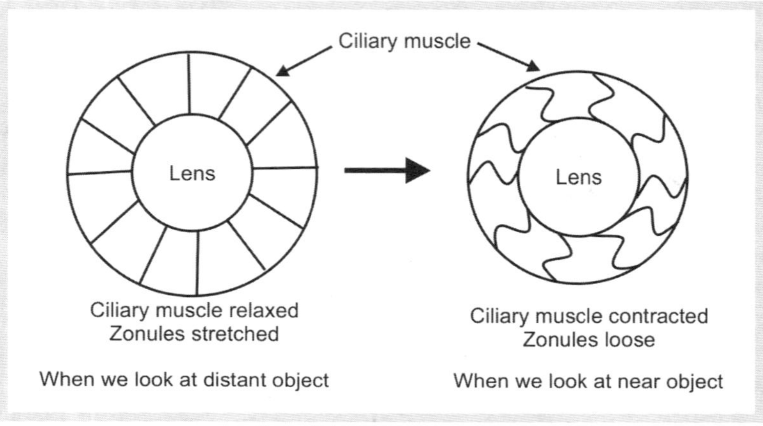

Fig. 7.1: Mechanism of accommodation.

century, when ciliary muscle contracts, zonules get relaxed and the natural lens assumes more rounded shape increasing its power for near vision. **Liebermann theory** suggests that the contraction of ciliary muscle pushes vitreous body forwards which in turn causes forward movement of lens and hence increase in its power for near vision. **Dynamic iris theory** proposes that it is not the ciliary muscle

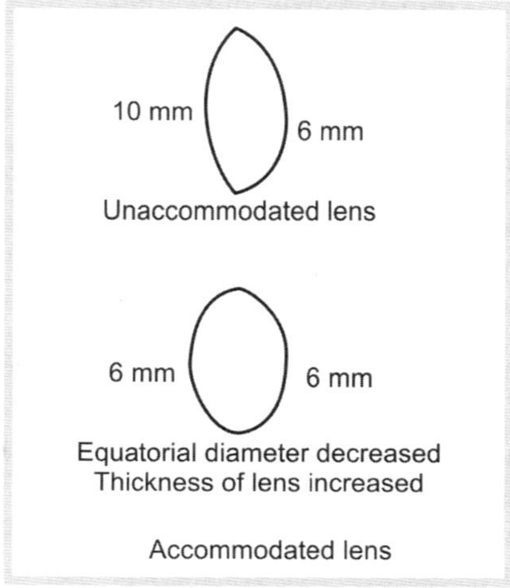

Fig. 7.2: Lateral view (MOA).

but the muscle of iris which when contracts, alters the anterior chamber depth and hence makes the lens change its shape and position. **Schachar and Fincham** also proposed mechanism of accommodation but Young Helmholtz theory is the most accepted one.

PRESBYOPIA

It is an anomaly of accommodation in which near point of eye recedes back due to loss of elasticity of lens with age.

Symptoms

Patient complains of difficulty in reading and writing but distant vision is good. He may have headache after doing near work or hold a reading paper at farther distance from eyes.

Treatment

Plus lens is given in form of glasses or contact lens to correct the error. Presbyopic LASIK laser surgery can also be done however glasses are the most commonly employed method. Power of lens depends on the age and working distance of patient as shown below:

40 + 1.00
45 + 1.50
50 + 2.00
55 + 2.50

60 or above +2.50: as the working distance is usually not nearer than 25 cm and the dioptric requirement for the distance of 25 cm is 2.50D.

Aphakia and Pseudophakia---+2.50DS to +3.00DS (in cases of compromised distant vision). If the best-corrected visual acuity (BCVA) does not improve up to 6/6 due to any reason like ARMD, +3.00DS or more near correction may be given to enable the patient read near letters.

Always bear in mind that near correction must be given after doing correction for distance. Both eyes should be checked individually and minimum possible correction should be given for near. Due consideration should be given to the profession and habits of the patient while fixing the near point.

Why Presbyopia Should be Slightly Undercorrected

When we read near objects accommodation and convergence both are required. Presbyopia is always undercorrected so as to encourage accommodation. Accommodation is accompanied by accommodative convergence. Thus, patients do not complain of eyestrain symptoms. Full correction of presbyopia causes eyestrain symptoms due to lack of accommodative convergence.

Pre-presbyopia: The usual age of beginning of presbyopia is considered to be 40 years, but in some patients, it may set in before the age of 40 years. This is also known as Early Presbyopia. In case, a patient finds difficulty in reading near targets before 40, he can be categorized as pre-presbyopic patient. But, ruling out the presence of uncorrected hyperopia for distance is a must. Diabetes and glaucoma must always be ruled out as both these conditions cause damage to ciliary muscle and patient complains of frequent change of glasses and early onset of presbyopia.

Accommodation insufficiency: It is closely related to presbyopia but exists in young population. The patient has symptoms of difficulty in near vision (more in cases of hyperopia), headache and eyestrain while working at near distance. It requires appropriate refraction for distance. The hyperopes are usually undercorrected whereas the myopes are slightly overcorrected in order to stimulate accommodation. In certain cases, mild addition of +0.50DS or +0.75DS is given for symptomatic relief.

Paralysis of Accommodation

This condition is known as cycloplegia. It may be caused by use of cycloplegic drugs like atropine, third nerve paralysis and internal ophthalmoplegia (paralysis of ciliary muscle and sphincter pupillae muscle). Patient complains of blurring of vision for near; less marked in myopic patients and intolerance to light due to associated dilatation of pupil. On examination pupil is dilated, light reflex is absent and range of accommodation is decreased. Treatment consists of removal of causative factor, prescription of plus lens for reading and dark goggles to avoid photophobia. Effect of drug weans off gradually of its own.

Spasm of accommodation: This is a condition in which ciliary muscle over contracts and patient exerts abnormally excessive accommodation. It may be caused by pilocarpine like drugs. Children with uncorrected refractive error sometimes go into spasm of accommodation in an effort to compensate for the refractive error. It may be associated with bad reading habits like poor illumination, bad posture, mental stress, etc. The shift to digital era has increased exposure to various digital devices and excessive near work. This is also one of the major reasons leading to spasm of accommodation. Patient complains of poor distance vision due to induced myopia and pain around eyes accompanied with other asthenopic symptoms. If dry refraction is done at this moment, myopic prescription will be given to the patient, which is incorrect. This is the reason that dry refraction should not be done in children. Refraction under appropriate cycloplegics will confirm the diagnosis. The patient is treated by giving atropine for a few weeks. He is advised to avoid reading for some time. Removal of associated causative factors such as poor illumination should also be taken care of.

Accommodation infacility: It may be a component of accommodation dysfunction, with other components being accommodation insufficiency (inadequate focusing ability) and accommodation excess (over-focusing). Patients suffering from accommodation infacility complain of difficulty in shifting its focus from far to near distance and vice-versa. For example: patient finds that the blackboard is blurry after long duration of near work and vice-versa. Exact cause of accommodation infacility is not clear but it appears that muscle weakness, prolonged near work, uncorrected refractive errors and underlying visual or neurological conditions may contribute to its development. For these patients, appropriate prescription is necessary along with accommodation exercises like The HART chart. HART chart is a vision chart designed for distance as well as near which allows the patient to alter their focus between distance and near.

CONVERGENCE

It is a type of binocular movement of eyeballs in which the two eyes simultaneously and synchronously turn inwards to provide binocular single vision for near. It may be voluntary or reflex. Reflex convergence is of four types:

1. **Proximal convergence:** Psychological awareness of a near object initiates this type of convergence.

2. **Tonic:** It means that when the patient is awake there is an inherent tone in the extra ocular muscles.
3. **Fusional:** It is initiated by a bi-temporal retinal image disparity and is not associated with change in refractive status of eyeball. It ensures that image of an object falls on corresponding retinal points in the two eyes.
4. **Accommodative:** It is initiated by act of accommodation. It means that when we accommodate; we converge. It is a part of near reflex. One diopter of accommodation is accompanied by 3–5 prism diopters of accommodative convergence and it remains fairly constant. Abnormalities of accommodative convergence are associated with squint.

AC/A ratio: It can be defined as accommodative convergence measured in prism diopters per unit change in accommodation measured in diopters. Normal value is 3–5 prism diopters. It means that with one diopter of accommodation there is 3–5 prism diopter of convergence. It decreases with age. It is calculated by different methods namely heterophoria and gradient method.

- **Heterophoria method:** Deviation of eyeball is measured in prism diopters with patient looking at 6 meters distance with full spectacle correction. This can be done by Maddox rod test or cover uncover test. Deviation is again measured with same optical correction with patient looking at an object kept at a distance of 33 cm using cover uncover technique. Interpupillary distance (IPD) is measured in cm with a scale. Now the AC/A ratio is calculated as:
  AC/A ratio = IPD + $(H_n - H_d)/D$
  Where,
  IPD = Interpupillary distance (in centimeters)
  H_n = Deviation for near (33 cm or 3 diopter) (in prism diopters)
  H_d = Deviation for distance at 6 meters (in prism diopters)
  D = Fixation Distance for near in **Diopters** (33 cm = 3 diopter)
  Note: Esodeviation is denoted in plus, whereas, exodeviation is denoted in minus.
- **Gradient method:** This method is based on the fact that if we put minus lenses in front of eye, they increase the requirement of accommodation and if we put plus lenses before eye, they relax accommodation. Further, it is assumed that 1DS lens is equivalent to 1D of accommodation.

First of all, deviation is measured at near with full optical correction. Now Plus 3 lens is put in front of full optical correction and again the deviation is measured for near. AC/A ratio is measured as follows:

- AC/A ratio: (Phoria with additional lenses—baseline phoria)/(Power of additional lenses)
- For example: Baseline phoria 2PD exophoria, with additional 3D plus lenses it is 14PD exophoria.
- AC/A ratio = 14 – 2/ 3 = 4:1
- Other methods for determining AC/A ratio are Fixation disparity method and haploscopic method.

Significance of AC/A ratio: A high AC/A ratio is associated with convergent squint when the patient sees a near object. There is no squint if the patient sees a distant object but when he sees a near object, there is convergent squint. It is treated by prescribing +3.00DS lens for near along with the correction of refractive error for distance if any, so that while seeing near objects he does not need to accommodate. Withdrawal of spectacles for near in a child with high AC/A ratio depends upon degree of hypermetropia, AC/A ratio and the amount of associated astigmatism. A low AC/A ratio is associated with divergent squint when patient sees a near object.

Convergence insufficiency: This is a condition which occurs more commonly in school going children. Patient complains of eyestrain symptoms while reading, working on computer and watching TV. There may or may not be associated refractive error. This is because when we look at near object we need to converge. If medial recti are not strong enough to sustain convergence it puts strain on eyes hence headache and other symptoms. It can be confirmed by testing range of fusion on synoptophore. If patient is not able to sustain 30° convergence, i.e., 6–10 cm proximity of near target with best possible correction he is diagnosed as a patient of convergence insufficiency. Treatment consists of convergence exercises after correction of refractive error if any and good nutrition.

Convergence excess: It is a condition in which the eye converges more than normal for each diopter of change in accommodation. Such patients might present with esodeviation, which is more for near as compared to distance. Appropriate refraction is necessary as convergence excess might be accompanied with accommodation anomalies. Full correction of hyperopia or under-correction of myopia can be used as a therapy along with prescription of prisms if patient complains of diplopia.

Near point of convergence (NPC): Closest point at which an object can be seen as a single object with both eyes open. If the object is brought nearer to NPC, patient will complain of diplopia.

Far point of convergence (FPC): It is a relative position of eyes when they are in resting position. It is usually infinity. At resting position, the two eyes may be slightly divergent hence the FPC may be negative means behind the eye.

Range of convergence: The distance between FPC and NPC is the range of convergence. The part of convergence that lies between the eye and the infinity is the positive convergence and the part that lies beyond infinity (behind the eye) is the negative convergence.

Amplitude of convergence: It is the difference in convergence power required to maintain the eyes in a position of rest and in a position of maximum convergence.

How to do Convergence Exercises?

Convergence exercises can be done at home or with the help of synoptophore. Exercise must be done after using spectacles, if any.

At Home

Hold a pencil or any pointed object at arm's length. See the tip of the object with both eyes. Start bringing the object closer to the eyes and maintain your focus at the tip of the object. When the object is close to eyes it will appear blurred or there might be doubling of tip of the object. Stop bringing further closer and try to focus the tip by converging your eyes. After some time the tip of the object appears clear and single. Bring the object still closer. Again the tip will get blurred, focus the tip again and repeat the procedure till you feel headache. At this point, close your eyes and rest for a few seconds. Bring the object back and again start bringing closer. This can be done for about ten minutes at one time or till the eyes get tired.

With Synoptophore

Put slides of fusion in the slot of synoptophore provided for the purpose. Bring the arms of the synoptophore at zero. Ask the patient to see the slides through eye piece. Patient sees a single image. Now converge the arms slightly and see whether the patient maintains fusion. If patient starts complaining that he is experiencing diplopia, ask him to make the image single by exercising his convergence capacity. When he again sees single image, further converge the arms of synoptophore. Again the patient will experience diplopia. Ask him to exercise his convergence capacity more and fuse the image. This goes on till his range of fusion becomes around 35°.

Retinoscopy and Transposition

RETINOSCOPY

This is also known as skiascopy or shadow test. It is an objective method for determination of refractive error by using principle of neutralization with accommodation at rest.

Types of Retinoscopy

It is of two types namely *wet and dry*. When retinoscopy is done with use of some drug it is called wet retinoscopy. When it is done without use of any drug it becomes dry retinoscopy. Wet retinoscopy has got certain advantages that accommodation is relaxed with the use of cycloplegic, fundus examination is done side-by-side and some hidden disease like primary open angle glaucoma, diabetic retinopathy can be detected early in its course and spasm of accommodation is relieved with the use of cycloplegic. The disadvantage is that patient has to come again for final prescription and he has to tolerate photophobia, chances of drug allergy, etc. Still wet retinoscopy is the best method.

Depending upon accommodation used it is further divided into two types; *static* retinoscopy when patient is looking at distant object and accommodation is at rest and *dynamic* retinoscopy when it is done with patient looking at near object and accommodation is being exercised. Dynamic retinoscopy is not of much significance.

Retinoscopes

They are of two types:

1. **Mirror retinoscopes:** This may be a plane mirror or concave mirror with a hole in the center. A combination of both plane and concave mirrors is also available known as Priestley-Smith mirror **(Fig. 8.1)**.

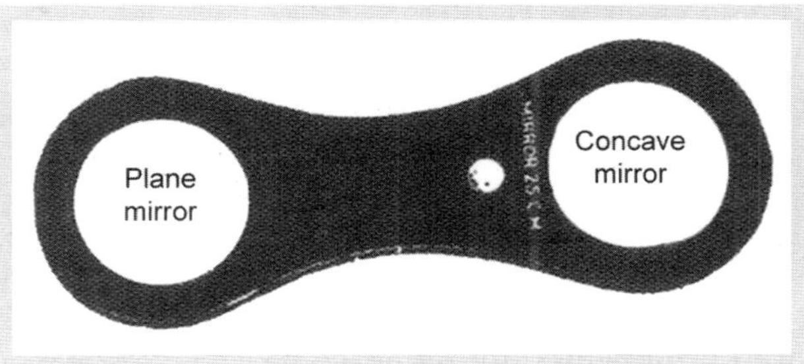

Fig. 8.1: Priestley-Smith mirror.

2. **Self-illuminated retinoscopes:** There is an inbuilt source of light in the retinoscope. These are further of two types—spot retinoscope and streak retinoscope. Streak retinoscope is more commonly employed as it is easy to detect axis of astigmatism with this mirror **(Fig. 8.2)**.

Principle

This is based on the principle that when light is reflected by a mirror into the eye of a person, the direction in which the light will travel across the pupil depends on the refractive status of the eyeball.

Procedure

It is done in a dark room with a retinoscope. Patient is seated at a distance of six meters from Snellen's chart and his visual acuity is recorded in both the eyes separately. Patient is asked to look at infinity so that his accommodation is relaxed. With the help of a spot or streak retinoscope light is thrown in his eyes one by one. We appreciate a red fundal glow in pupillary area. Move the retinoscope up and down, right and left and notice the movement of glow. There are three possibilities (with plane mirror retinoscope):

1.	Glow moves with the movement of retinoscope	Emmetropia, hypermetropia and myopia less than 1.00 D
2.	Glow moves against the movement of retinoscope	Myopia more than 1.00 D
3.	Glow does not show any movement	Myopia 1.00 D

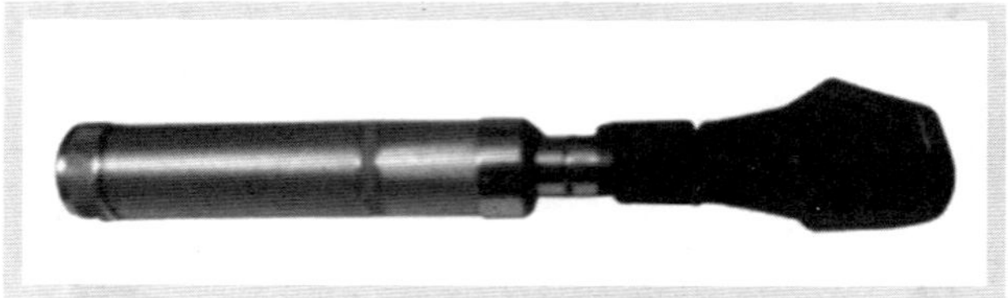

Fig. 8.2: Streak retinoscope.

If concave mirror is used for retinoscopy, e.g., in hazy media the interpretations are as follows:

1.	Glow moves with the movement of retinoscope	Myopia more than 1.00 D
2.	Glow moves against the movement of retinoscope	Emmetropia, hypermetropia and myopia less than 1.00 D
3.	Glow does not show any movement	Myopia 1.00 D

Now if the glow shows with movement with plane mirror retinoscope, add plus lens till the glow stops moving with the movement of retinoscope and add minus lens if glow shows against movement till there is no movement. This is the point of neutralization. Note down the power of lens required to neutralize the movement of glow. This is the retinoscopy reading. Note down the distance between the patient and the observer. Movement of glow is fast if error is of small degree and it is slow when error is of high degree.

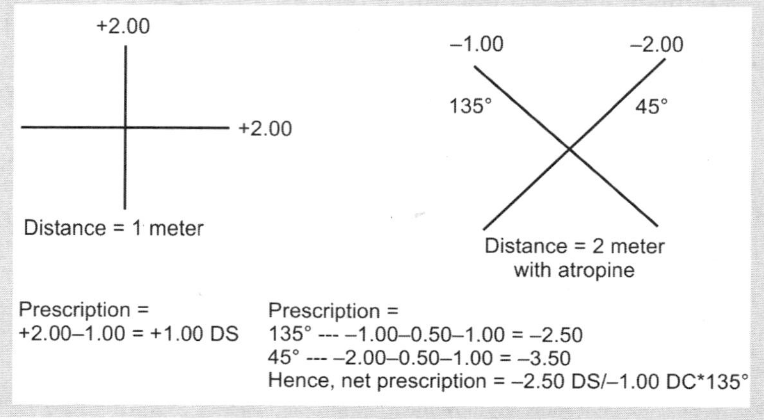

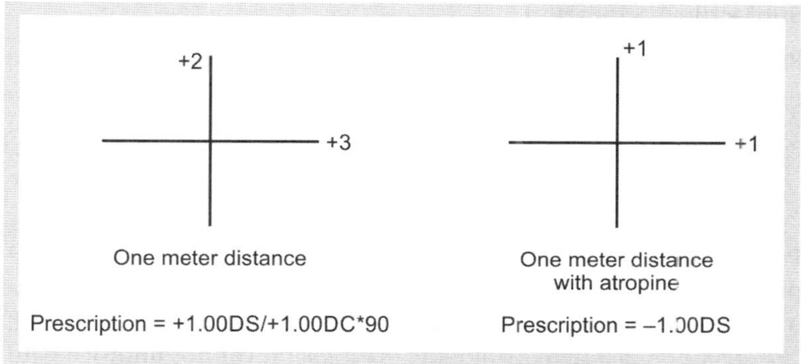

Distance factor = 100/distance between patient and observer in cm.

For example: Distance factor for one meter distance = 100/100 cm = 1
Distance factor for half meter distance = 100/50 = 2
Distance factor for two meter distance = 100/200 = 0.5

Drugs Used in Retinoscopy

Retinoscopy done after using drugs is known as wet retinoscopy and retinoscopy done without drugs is known as dry retinoscopy. Atropine should be used in children less than 5-year-old. Homatropine should be used between ages of 5 to 15 years. Cyclopentolate can also be used. These are cycloplegic drugs (paralyze ciliary muscle and accommodation is relaxed). Tropicamide and phenylephrine or combination of both can be used in adult patients. Effect of atropine lasts for one to two weeks, homatropine for 3 to 4 days, Cyclopentolate for 1 to 2 days and Tropicamide/phenylephrine for 3 to 4 hours. During this period patient finds difficult to do near work and complains of photophobia. So these side effects should be explained to the patient before putting eye drops in his eyes.

Drug Factor

Atropine = 1
Homatropine = 0.5
Cyclopentolate = 0.5
Other drugs = none

Now deduct the distance factor and drug factor from the retinoscopy findings. This gives the objective prescription for the patient.

Subjective Verification

Put the lens of desired power as per the objective findings and ask the patient to read. Increase or decrease the power of lens by ±0.25 DS. Prescribe the power of lens with which patient can read the best in terms of visual acuity and comfort.

Confirmation of Subjective Refraction

Pinhole test: Pinhole is placed in front of prescribed glasses and patient is asked to read Snellen's chart. If visual acuity improves with pinhole, it means still some minor error needs to be corrected. However, if it is a high astigmatic error vision cannot improve with glasses beyond a particular limit but still it improves with pinhole. However, if vision decreases after using pinhole it means some opacity is present in the medium like central corneal opacity, posterior subcapsular cataract, etc.

Duochrome test: It is based on chromatic aberration. In an emmetropic person rays of light are focused on retina. As we know that white light is made up of seven colors namely Violet, Indigo, Blue, Green, Yellow, Orange, and Red (VIBGYOR). All colors have got different wavelength so they are focused at different points on retina. Red color with maximum wavelength is focused behind the retina, green color in front of retina and yellow color on retina. Thus an emmetropic person sees red and green colors equally sharp. After giving correction patient is asked to read "FRIEND". The FIN letters are written in green and RED letters are written in red color. If myopia is over corrected or hypermetropia is under corrected patient will appreciate green letters much better than red letters. On the other hand if myopia is under corrected or hypermetropia is over corrected patient will appreciate red color much better. Accordingly change in power of lens should be done so that the patient appreciates green and red letters equally sharp **(Fig. 8.3A)**.

FIN appears better than RED	Overcorrected myopia or under corrected hypermetropia
RED appears better than FIN	Overcorrected hypermetropia or under corrected myopia

Jackson's cross cylinder: It is used to verify power and axis of a cylindrical prescription. First of all verify power of a sphere if any by some other method. Then verify power of cylinder followed by axis

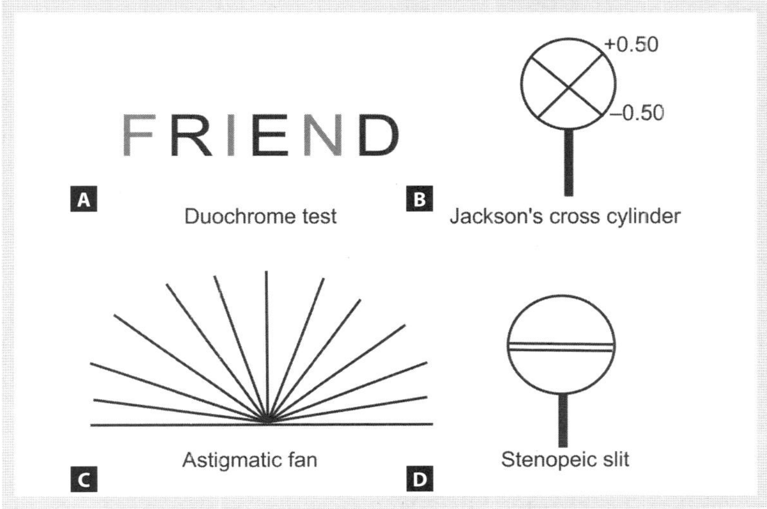

Figs. 8.3A to D: Methods for verification of subjective acceptance.

of cylinder by using JCC. The JCC is available in powers of 0.50 D or 0.25 D. Any of them can be used. For confirmation of power of cylinder place the JCC with axis along the axis of prescribed cylinder and ask the patient which one is better. Now place the JCC in reverse order and again ask which one is better. If prescription is correct patient should see better without JCC. If however one of the positions of JCC is better, increase or decrease the power of cylinder prescribed and repeat the test till patient sees better without JCC. For confirmation of axis place the JCC in such a way that the two axis of JCC make an angle of 45° with axis of prescribed cylinder. If patient sees better with JCC rotate the axis of plus cylinder towards plus axis of JCC and minus cylinder towards minus axis of JCC till he sees better without JCC **(Fig. 8.3B)**.

Astigmatic fan test: It consists of a dial of radiating lines at an interval of 10°. Patient is given best suitable combination of lenses and asked to look at the astigmatic fan with one eye closed. A person with no astigmatism sees all the lines equally clear. An astigmatic person sees one line more sharply defined than the others. Now add +0.50 DS lens over and above the best combination of lenses already given. This causes fogging. Now add concave cylinder at axis right angle to the axis of clearest line visible on astigmatic fan. Power of cylinder should be such that all lines are equally sharp **(Fig. 8.3C)**.

Stenopeic slit: It is used to verify axis and strength of cylinder. After doing retinoscopy and subjective acceptance spherical correction is put in the trial frame. Ask the patient to read with one eye closed. Slit is put in the trial frame and rotated till the patient sees the clearest vision. This is the axis of the cylinder required. Now put some spherical power which gives the best vision with slit still in place. Note down the power of this spherical (suppose –0.50 DS and slit is at 45°). Rotate the slit by 90° and again put the spherical power till it gives the best vision. Again note down this power (suppose –1.50 DS with slit at 135°). Now the algebraic difference of two spherical powers, i.e., –0.50 and –1.50 (–1.00 DS) is the power of cylinder required at 45° **(Fig. 8.3D)**.

Difficulties Faced during Retinoscopy

- **Glow is not visible:** This may be because of hazy media due to corneal opacity, cataract or vitreous opacity. Dilate the pupil and confirm the diagnosis by slit lamp examination.
- **Movement of glow cannot be appreciated:** It may be due to high refractive errors. Put +10.00 DS or –10.00 DS lens and notice the glow.
- **Scissor shadow:** This difficulty is faced with dilated pupil. Constrict the pupil and do retinoscopy.
- **Conflicting shadows:** Different shadows are seen moving in different directions. This is seen in irregular astigmatism. It cannot be corrected by prescribing glasses. Semisoft contact lens need to be prescribed.
- **Triangular shadow:** It is seen in keratoconus. Semisoft contact lens need to be prescribed.
- **Changing retinoscopy findings:** It happens if the patient is accommodating. Ask the patient to look at infinity or paralyze the accommodation with a suitable drug.

TRANSPOSITION

It means making equivalent forms of prescription. It is required:

- For manufacturing of glasses.
- Sometimes refractive error of a patient needs plus cylinder at 90° in one eye and minus cylinder at 90° in other eye. In such cases we

make the power of cylinder plus or minus in both the eyes to avoid eyestrain. This is possible by transposition only.

- Glass in a frame is always fitted in a curved manner. This curve introduces a definite power in the glass. This is called base curve of glass. To neutralize this undesired power; transposition is mandatory in all cases.

Simple Transposition

It is done by observing following rules:

- Power of new sphere is calculated by algebraic sum of power of given sphere and power of given cylinder.
- Change the sign of given cylinder keeping power same.
- Rotate the axis of given cylinder by 90°.

Examples: **+1.00 DS/+0.50 DC × 90°**
Power of new sphere = +1.00+ (+0.50) = +1.50 DS
Power of new cylinder = 0.50 DC with opposite sign (minus) and axis 180°.

Thus the new prescription becomes +1.50 DS/–0.50 DC × 180. This is called simple transposition.

Toric Transposition

For toric transposition a base curve is required. The following rules should be observed for toric transposition:

- Sign of cylinder should be same as sign of base curve. If not change the sign of cylinder by doing simple transposition.
- Power of new sphere = Power of given sphere minus power of base curve.
- Power of cylinder no 1 = Power of base curve with same sign and axis rotated by 90°.
- Power of cylinder no 2 = Power of given cylinder + power of base curve with same axis as of given cylinder.

Example: **–2.00 DS/–0.50 DC × 90° Base Curve + 5.00**
Rule No 1: Sign of cylinder should be same as sign of base curve. Sign of cylinder needs to be changed by simple transposition.
–2.50 DS/+0.50 DC × 180°
Rule no 2: Power of new sphere= –2.50 – (+5.00) = –7.50 DS
Rule no 3: Power of cylinder no 1 = +5.00 DC × 90°
Rule no 4: Power of cylinder no 2 = + 0.50 DC + (+5.00 DC) = + 5.50 DC × 180°

Thus the new prescription becomes
–7.50 DS/(+5.00 DC × 90°)(+5.50 DC × 180°)
Some Examples of Transposition

Example 1: +1.00 DS/+3.00 DC × 90° Base curve of –6.00
Hence + 4.00 DS /–3.00 DS × 180° Base curve of –6.00
Net prescription will be:
+10.00 DS/(–6.00 DC × 90°)(–9.00 DC × 180°)

Example 2: –2.00 DS/–1.00 DC × 145° Base curve of –6.00
Net prescription will be:
+4.00 DS/(–6.00 DC × 55°)(–7.00 DC × 145°)

A Practical Problem

Suppose a patient has been prescribed +2.00 DS/–1.00 DC × 180° both eyes with add for near +2.50 DS both eyes. Patient wants glasses to be made for distance and near separately. What will be the prescription for near and distance glasses? Answer to this problem is that the patient should be prescribed +2.00 DS/–1.00 DC × 180° both eyes for distance and +4.50 DS/–1.00 DC × 180° for near. Point to be remembered is that '*add*' is algebraically added to the spherical power for distance and there is no change in power and axis of cylinder.

How to make a Cross Cylinder of Power 0.50?

Make a glass of –0.50 DS/+1.00 DC × 180°. Power of spherical should be half of power of cylinder with opposite signs.

9

CHAPTER

Ophthalmic Lenses

TYPES OF OPHTHALMIC LENS MATERIALS

Different types of materials are available for making ophthalmic lenses. They are:

Glass

This has been the most commonly used lens material. It is colorless, transparent, resistant to heat and scratch with good optical qualities. It is available as Crown glass (refractive index 1.523) and Flint (ref. index 1.650). Glasses of higher refractive indices are thinner and lighter than glasses of lower refractive indices, so more suitable material for high power lenses.

Photochromatic lenses darken on exposure to light and become colorless in the dark again. This is because silver chloride crystals are incorporated in the glass material, which on exposure to sunlight become darker in color. Glasses are also available in different tints, which is a permanent feature.

Chemical treatment, lamination or heat treatment makes the lens impact resistant. Chemical treatment is the best method as it gives optically good quality glasses.

Plastic Lenses or Resin Lenses

These lenses are popularly known as fiber lenses or plastic lenses. They are transparent, break-resistant, impact-resistant, lightweight with good optical qualities but prone to scratches and more costly than glass lenses. Most commonly used material is CR-39 (C stands for Columbia and R stands for resin). This material can withstand heat up to 100 °C. Its refractive index is 1.498. Chemically, it is allyl diglycol carbonate. Tints can be easily applied and changed if required later on. It is UV-absorbing lens so protects against ultraviolet radiations.

Resin lenses of higher refractive index are also available suitable for high power lenses. One can easily appreciate that if you come out of air-conditioned environment, there occurs fogging of spectacle lenses. This fogging of lenses in response to change in environment is less in resin lenses as compared to glass lenses. These lenses can be made scratch resistant by a special type of coating over the lens. They are also thicker than glass lenses so the edge of concave lenses becomes prominent.

Polycarbonate Lenses

This material is heat sensitive hence can crack in hot or cold environment, but highly impact resistant, thinnest and lightweight but prone to scratches. A special scratch-resistant coating is required. Vision around edges is distorted. Its refractive index is 1.586 thus thinner than resin lenses. It blocks both UVA and UVB rays. Tinting of these lenses is difficult. Due to their impact resistance, these lenses are suitable for stuntmen and sportspersons, persons involved in hazardous industries, children and single-eyed patients.

V-value Constringence or Abbe's Number

The degree to which the material has the same refractive index for different wavelengths of light. Lenses made with lower V values more quickly show rainbows, color fringes and degradation of best acuity when the eye turns towards the periphery of a spectacle lens, the effect being proportional to the power of lens. In simple language, it is a positive value that indicates the degree of transverse chromatic aberration. High V-value means low dispersive power and vice versa. Thus, crown glass has V-value of 59 and CR-39 has V-value of 57.8 and thus patient does not complain of colored fringes due to their low dispersive power. In contrast, high-index lenses and polycarbonate lenses have a low V-value thus high dispersive power and cause colored fringing of objects.

GRINDING OF LENSES

It is a procedure by which we convert a slab of glass (blank) into a spectacle lens with specific power. It is also known as *surfacing*. This is done by grinding the blank in such a way that curvatures are produced on both front and back surfaces. The difference of curvatures on both surfaces gives us the dioptric power of the lens. A wide range of tools calibrated for a specific power are required. These tools are made from cast iron and should be checked from time to time for their accuracy. Various processes involved in the making of lenses are as under **(Fig. 9.1)**.

- **Blocking:** It is a process by which a blank is fixed to the grinding machine. Gluing material is heated and applied between the blank and the platform of grinding machine. Once the material cools down; it holds the lens very tightly and grinding can be carried out easily.
- **Roughing:** It means generating the desired curvature. Surface of the blank is rotated against tool of specific curvature using sand or carborundum as abrasive powder. Thus, a blank is converted into a curved piece of glass with rough surface having approximate desired power.
- **Smoothening:** Here a proper tool with specific power is used to give accurate power to the blank. Fine abrasive material like aluminous oxide is used to grind the blank. Two grades of abrasive 302 and 303 are used one by one. Surface of the blank is trued with 302 and then with 303 to make it smoother. The end product of this process is the lens with correct power. It is ready for polishing.
- **Polishing:** A soft pad of felt cloth or wool cloth or specially designed polishing pads are attached to the tool of rough use.
- **Deblocking:** Polished lens is examined under incandescent bulb and if found satisfactory, the lens is deblocked from the metal block. The lens and the block are immersed in cold water and the block is tapped by a wooden mallet. Ice cubes may also be used to facilitate the deblocking process. Lens is cleaned with a thinner to remove any undesired particle over it.

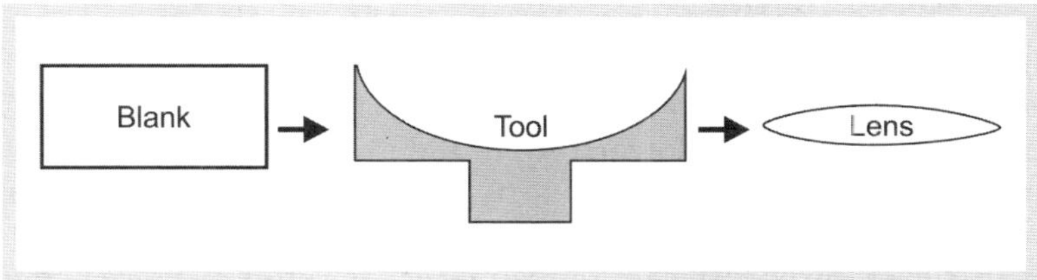

Fig. 9.1: Grinding of lens.

This process is repeated on the other surface of the lens. After each step lens and the block are cleaned properly, thickness of the lens is controlled during grinding of other surface.

BEST-FORM LENSES

An ideal lens should be free from all types of optical aberrations. The most important is that when we look through a lens obliquely, there should not be any aberration. A lens form which eliminates all these aberrations is known as best-form lens. One can easily understand that for different types of lens powers different types of base curves are required to achieve very good results. But practically this is not possible as it requires a huge stock of lenses and tools. Thus, we rely upon certain standard base curves. These base curves are:

From +7D to Plane	Base curve of –6.00D is given on back surface
From 0 to -6D	Base curve of +6.00D on front surface
From -7D to –10D	Base curve of +3.00D on front surface
From -10D to –15D	Base curve of +1.25D on front surface
From -15D to –20D	Plano front surface

A lens with a base curve of 6D is known as *deep meniscus lens* and with a base curve of 1.25D is known as *Periscopic lens.*

Minus base curve is ground on back surface for making up to +7.00D lenses and a decreasing plus base curve is ground on the front surface ranging from +6D to plano for making of up to –20D lenses. Beyond +7D to –20D powers, it is not possible to neutralize the oblique astigmatism of lenses. However, with newer techniques and advent of computers for mathematical calculations it is possible to manufacture lenses of the best forms and services have become personalized.

PANTOSCOPIC TILT

It is the angle between the plane of the lens/frame front and frontal plane of the face. Upper 180° of eye wire is farther from the frontal plane of face and the lower 180° of the eye wire is nearer to the frontal plane of face. This is about 10–12°. This is required for proper relationship of frame front and the eyebrows/cheeks of patient's face. It also gives the widest view for reading as the vertex distance of the lower half of lens is minimized.

However, this tilt introduces some astigmatism and changes the effective power of the lens.

If the tilt is made in such a way that the upper 180° of frame comes closure to the frontal plane of face as compared to the lower 180°, it is called the retroscopic tilt.

TYPES OF LENSES

Single Vision Lenses (Monofocal)

The lenses which have same power throughout the entire surface of the lens are called single vision lenses. These lenses are used when the same prescription is used for distance and near both, e.g., young persons below the age of 40 years. They are also used when presbyopic patients require correction only for near vision or patient is not comfortable with bifocal prescription and wants to use spectacles for distance and near made separately.

Bifocal Lenses

Depending on design, they are of different types **(Fig. 9.2)**:
- Kryptok bifocal lenses
- Straight bifocal or executive bifocal lenses
- D-bifocal lenses
- Moon-shaped bifocal lenses
- Round bifocal lenses

Depending on manufacturing technique, they may be of different types:
- **Split bifocal:** It is also known as two-piece bifocal. Here two separate pieces of glass of different power are held together in a frame.
  This bifocal was invented by Benjamin Franklin. It is no more used nowadays.
- **Cemented bifocal:** A small plus lens is glued to the back of a distance prescription with a glue like Canada balsam which has the same refractive index as glass. This is used today in some low vision prescriptions which require very high additions.
  The modern variant of the cemented bifocal is the Fresnel lens which sticks in place with water or alcohol. It is used sometimes as a temporary bifocal, but it is cosmetically unappealing, expensive, and optically poor, hence not fit for permanent use.
- **Fused bifocal:** This is the most commonly used variety. Here a piece of glass of higher power with higher refractive index

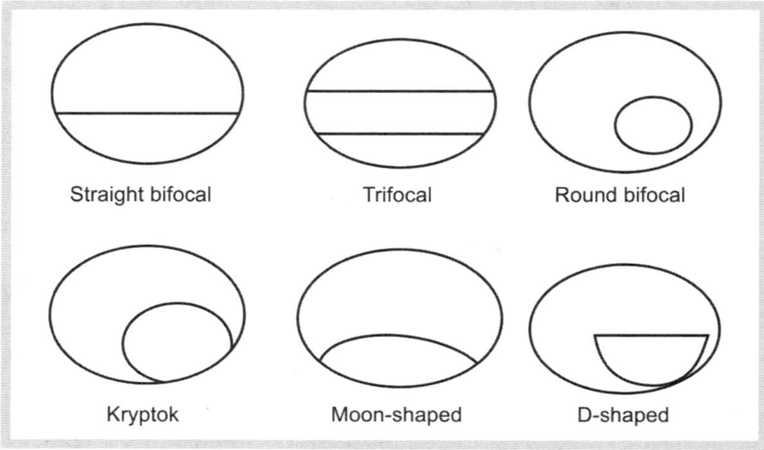

Fig. 9.2: Types of bifocal lenses.

(flint glass) is fused on the surface of crown glass. This part acts as segment for near vision. It has a good cosmetic appearance as there is no visible or palpable demarcation. An example of this type is Kryptok which means hidden in Latin.

A countersink curve is made on the front surface of crown glass with refractive index of 1.523. A button of flint glass with refractive index 1.65 with same curvature is prepared and fused on the countersink of crown glass at very high temperature of above 650°C. Since the ref. index of flint glass is higher, hence a round-shaped segment can be seen on the front surface without any palpable demarcation. Size of this round segment is between 22–26 mm. If any cylindrical power needs to be ground on the lens, it must be done on the back surface of the lens.

- **Solid bifocal:** This type of bifocal lens is made from a single material but different segments are ground with different curvatures. The line between the two segments is visible but can be made to disappear by joining the two segments with a transition zone. This is also known as one piece or seamless solid bifocals.

Trifocal Lenses

This lens has three segments for distance, intermediate (e.g., for computer) and near with different powers. Intermediate segment is 6–8 mm. This lens is no more used these days.

PROGRESSIVE ADDITION LENS

Progressive addition lens (PAL) lens is made with power for distance at the top of lens and power for near at the bottom of lens and there is a gradual transition of power from distance to near in the intermediate segment but no line is visible so gives better cosmetic appearance. A person using PAL can view the distant objects from the topmost segment, can do computer work from the intermediate segment and do his reading work from the bottom segment. This type of lens is particularly useful for persons who need to read and type and at the same time deal with public means who need to work at near, intermediate and far distance at the same time, e.g., officers working in banks need to read the cheque no. type it and confirm on monitor and at the same time deal with the public. The presence of a bifocal segment is taken as a sign of old age so a PAL without a demarcation appears more youthful.

The disadvantage is that periphery of lens has unwanted astigmatism hence not good for vision, thus eye movements are restricted. These lenses are costly and not affordable for every person. Fitting of lens requires special care. The optical center of lens must match the pupillary center to avoid difficulty in adjustment, on axis blur and the need to adopt uncomfortable head positions. Another point to be noted in the prescription of PAL is that the frame chosen should be of good vertical height otherwise there will be a problem in adjustment. Difficulty faced by small vertical height frame is that the patient has to move his head back and forth to see clearly on a monitor. This is described as moving one's head back and forth as if he is watching a tennis match. This is particularly important if the addition required is higher like +2.00DS or more. Problems faced by a beginner during adjustment period are headache and dizziness. Answer to this adjustment problem is removing the lens for some time and reusing it again once the symptoms are over.

The *Varilux* lens was the first PAL of modern design. It was developed by Bernard Maitenaz and patented in 1953.

Designs of PAL Lenses

There are different designs of PAL lenses. They are monodesign and multidesign, asymmetry and symmetry design, and hard and soft design. In multidesign the position for near vision segment goes up as the power of addition increases. This is because a patient holds the reading material nearer if the addition is higher. This is not the case with monodesign hence it is considered of inferior quality. In symmetrical PAL design right and left lenses are identical. Lenses have to be rotated 10° anticlockwise in right eye and 10°clockwise in left eye for nasal decentration of near segments. This causes uneven peripheral optical features and difficulty in adjustment. Asymmetrical PAL design lenses are made separate for right and left eyes hence no need for lens rotation. This results in better optical performance, better BSV and convergence and improved visual comfort. In hard design PAL, there is small intermediate zone (called small corridor), wide distance and near zones. It is difficult to adapt. Unwanted cylindrical power is pushed towards center of the lens therefore intermediate and peripheral visions are restricted. In soft PAL design distance and near zones are relatively smaller and intermediate zone is wider (called long corridor). Power changes gradually from distance to near. Unwanted cylinder power is pushed towards the periphery. Further modifications are being done to minimize adaptive problems with PAL lenses **(Fig. 9.3)**.

Bifocal, trifocal and progressive lenses should be better avoided in old patients who are using glasses for the first time and particularly if the addition for near is considerable. This is because there is a considerable problem while looking down and climbing down the stairs. This problem is doubled up in patients suffering from vertigo

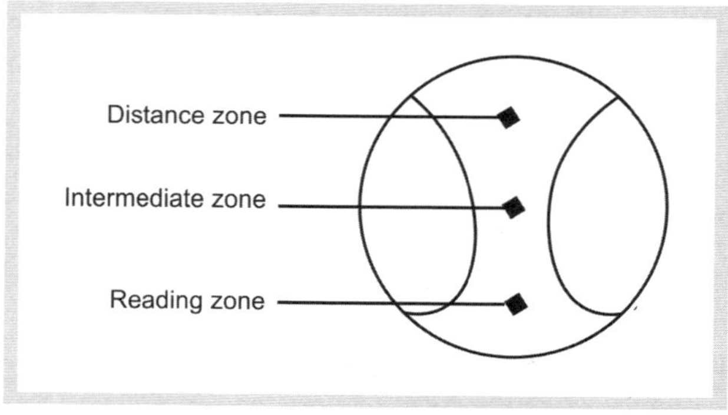

Fig. 9.3: Progressive addition lens (PAL).

and there are high chances of patient falling down. A separate pair of glasses for distance and near vision is ideal for them.

Markings of Progressive Addition Lenses

PALs consist of two types of markings:

1. **Temporary markings include:**
   - *Distance reference circle:* It contains the distance prescription.
   - *Fitting cross:* Point which centers in front of the pupil.
   - *Prism reference point:* It marks the beginning of the corridor of the lens.
   - *Near reference circle:* It contains the near prescription.

   All these markings are removed after the fitting of lenses.
2. **Permanent markings:** Also known as microetchings. These include laser marks which depict add power on temporal side of the lens and logo of the product on nasal side of the lens. These are visible only when focused against the light.

In case of first-time wearers, following instructions need to be given in order to promote adaptability:

- Make sure the frame sets appropriately on the face and behind the ear to ensure clear vision.
- Initially, wear the spectacles for a short duration of time and adapt to various zones of vision, i.e., distance, near and intermediate.
- While walking, the floor ahead needs to be seen through distance portion and avoid viewing through near portion.
- The sides of the lens have blurry vision due to its construction. In case, the patient wants to view on the sides, he is expected to turn his head in that direction. For example, while driving if one wants to see on the sides, he has to turn his head in that direction to get clarity.
- Take some time so that you get adapted to the progressive lenses before you drive a vehicle or step up or step down a stair with progressive lenses.

Troubleshooting of Progressive Lenses

In cases of progressive lenses, the patients can report complaints. Each complaint has its own cause and solution. Most common complaints are as follows:

Sl. No	Complaint	Cause	Solution
1.	Difficulty in distance vision	• Inappropriate distance refraction • Ill-fitted lenses • High-fitted lenses	• Appropriate refraction • Review prescription of lenses • Widening of nose bridge • Refit lenses
2.	Difficulty in near vision	• Inappropriate near refraction • Ill-fitted lenses • Low-fitted lenses • Inappropriate pantoscopic tilt	• Appropriate refraction • Review prescription of lenses • Narrowing of nose bridge • Change pantoscopic tilt of frame • Refit lenses

ANTIREFLECTIVE COATING

This coating is used to avoid glare faced by computer users and night drivers. When a ray of light strikes our glass of spectacles most of it enters the medium of glass but some of it is reflected back from air-glass interface which creates glare, i.e., the object appears less sharp. This problem causes trouble to persons who work on computers for long hours and drive at night.

Antireflective coating works on the principle of destructive interference, i.e., when two light waves meet in such a way that the crest of one wave falls on trough of other wave (180°out of phase), they cancel out each other. Glass is coated with a special type of coating in such a way that the light reflected from air-coating interface and coating-glass interface forms destructive interference as shown in **Figure 9.4**.

AR coating is done on both the surfaces of lens, i.e., front and back surface to avoid glare from both the surfaces of lens. It is a multilayered coating which can be done on almost all types of glasses.

Material (dielectric) for coating is chosen in such a way that its refractive index is equal to the square root of the refractive index of spectacle lens and thickness of coating material is one-fourth of wavelength of light. Now because white light is a combination of different wavelengths hence multiple coatings are required to prevent reflection of light.

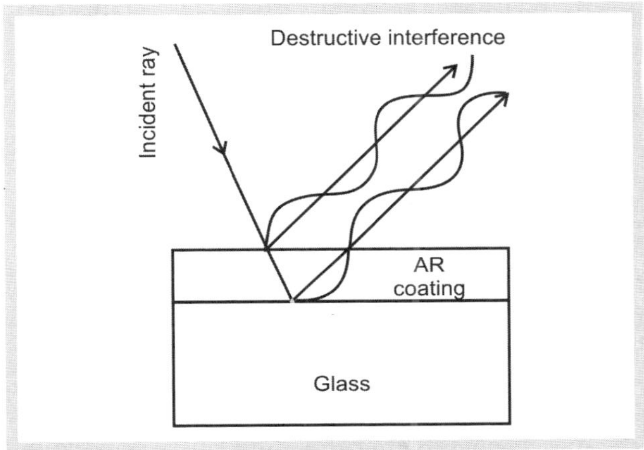

Fig. 9.4: Antireflective (AR) coating.

Advantages

It improves optical performance of lens, i.e., the wearer sees better and looks better with AR-coated glass. As maximum light passes through the lens, it improves contrast. It is very useful in persons who drive at night and use computers for long hours.

TINTING OF LENSES

This is done to decrease transmission of light through lens by making it appear colored. These lenses are used to avoid bright sunlight and sometimes for cosmetic reasons.

Different colors and shades are available for this purpose. Shades are usually expressed as a number or percentage. The percentage indicates the percentage of light transmission blocked. Persons using tinted glasses are advised not to drive at night.

Some Important Facts about Tinting

- Tint is a permanent feature in glass lenses. It cannot be changed. In resin lenses, tint can be darkened or lightened. However, if a light tinted resin lens is darkened, scratches on it become more prominent.
- It does not change its color from light to dark if exposed to sunlight.

- Polycarbonate lenses can also be lightened or darkened but with more difficulty.
- Tints cause more reflection and transmission of light is decreased.
- A plane lens where thickness of center and periphery is equal, tint appears uniform. However, in convex lens tint is more prominent in the center and in concave lens it is more prominent at the periphery.
- Special care has to be taken if the refractive error on two sides is significantly different.
- Tinted lenses attract dust and debris, hence need cleaning more frequently.
- Red, green and yellow tints should not be used as they interfere with traffic signal interpretation.
- If both antireflective coating and tinting are required, tinting has to be done first.
- Silver or chromium coating can be applied on lenses to give the effect of mirror coating so that the patient can see everything but passersby cannot see his eyes.
- Tint can be applied in a uniform manner over the whole lens or in a gradient manner. In gradient manner, the top of the lens is tinted the darkest and gradually faded to clear at the bottom.
- The smaller the lens, the lesser are the color shade variations.

Technique of Tinting Lenses

- **Surface coating:** A deposit material is coated on the back surface of the lens to increase surface reflections. This method is used to tint glass lenses.
- **Dye tinting:** Resin lenses are tinted by this method. Lens is kept in a dye chamber bath. The dye penetrates the lens material. Polycarbonate lenses are difficult to tint. However, the hard coat over polycarbonate lenses takes up the tint.
- **Solid glass tint:** Here the material of the glass itself is being tinted by adding some special chemical to the raw material of the lenses. Different tints available in the market are:

A1 = Light blue	A2 = Deep blue	B1 = Light gray
B2 = Deep gray	SP2 = Light pink	SP4 = Deep pink
SP9 = Light brown	SP10 = Deep brown	

Significance of Different Colors

Pink color is cosmetically better because it blends well with the skin tones. Grey color is considered cool sunglass color. Brown color is taken as warm cosmetic color. Yellow color is used during skiing, hunting and shooting to enhance target definition. It enhances contrast during cloudy and foggy weather.

Tinted lenses for outdoor use should be incorporated with ultraviolet absorbing material to avoid damage to retina. *While indoor,* tinted lenses should be such that they absorb blue color and transmit most of other colors. This is because while working under fluorescent bulb, flickering of light is there and it is maximum near blue end of spectrum. Blocking of flicker reduces incidence of headache. *While driving,* tint should not interfere with traffic signals.

PHOTOCHROMISM

Photochromic lens changes its color according to light and dark conditions.

It becomes dark in bright sunlight and again light colored in dim light conditions. This is because such lenses contain microscopically trapped silver chloride crystals which change into free silver on exposure to sunlight. This free silver forms silver colloids which absorb UV radiations to cause darkening of lenses. In indoor conditions, silver particles combined with trapped halides and silver halide crystals are reformed and lens appears clear.

Photochromatic lenses are available in glass, polycarbonate and plastic lenses. Corning was the first to manufacture glass photochromic lenses in 1960s. American Optical Association first introduced plastic photochromatic lenses in 1980s but it was successful in 1991 when Transitions Optical introduced them. These lenses darken only in sunlight but not in artificial light because UV radiations are required for the darkening effect. Hence car windows which block UV rays also render these lenses less effective inside the car.

Photochromic lenses should always be replaced in pairs so that there is no difference of shade in the two lenses. Old photochromic lens has undergone many light/dark cycles hence its color will be darker as compared to new photochromic lens. All photochromic lenses have additional UV absorbing property. Time taken by a photochromic lens to become dark in sunlight is less than time taken to clear again in indoor conditions.

Photochromic lenses absorb only UV light. Thus, they are not protective against infrared rays. These lenses become dark on exposure to UV light hence this may happen even in a room. Darkening performance is poor on a foggy day. Color change is temperature dependent. They become darker in winters than in summers. Photochromic lenses are slightly thicker than other lenses. The more is the thickness, the more is the darkening effect. These lenses show their optimum darkening effect after 10 dark/light cycles. The more they are exposed to sunlight, the darker they become. Glass photochromic lenses are available in grey and brown shades.

Photochromism in glass lenses is temperature dependent. They become darker in cold climate and clear easily in hot summers. So they are more suitable for snow skiers than beach goers while outside.

Technique

Technique of photochromism in resin lenses is much more difficult. Photosensitive molecules of indolino spironaphthoxazine are uniformly distributed within the front surface of the lens up to a depth of 100–150 micrometer. These lenses are also temperature sensitive. This lens becomes darker in cold temperature. Corning photochromic lenses are also available in which photosensitive material is present within the substance of the resin lens. So they have much longer life like glass lenses.

When exposed to light, photochromic lenses darken substantially in response to UV light in less than one minute and then continue to darken slightly over the next fifteen minutes. The lenses will begin to clear as soon as they are away from UV light, and will be noticeably lighter within two minutes and mostly clear within five minutes. However, it normally takes more than fifteen minutes for the lenses to completely fade to their nonexposed state.

Advantages and Disadvantages

Photochromatic lenses are never entirely transparent. They do not darken in artificial light. However, they protect against UV light and are useful for patients who are sensitive to light.

Effect of AR Coating on Photochromism

AR coating decreases reflection of incident light on lens and increases its transmittance. As the AR coating absorbs ultraviolet rays hence less light is available for activation of photochromic property of lens. Thus, a photochromic lens with AR coating becomes less dark on exposure to light as compared to a normal photochromic lens.

SCRATCH RESISTANT OR HARD COATING

This is a very thin coating done over resin lenses and polycarbonate lenses to protect them from scratches. However, it cannot protect them from scratches from very hard and sharp objects. It also protects tints and AR coating. Optical effect of this coating is negligible as the refractive index of this coating and lens material is almost same.

Hard coat may be applied on one or both surfaces of lens. Usually, these coatings are very long-lasting. Tinting of resin lenses becomes difficult after hard coating. Hard coating also increases antireflective properties hence transmittance of light is increased.

WATER-RESISTANT COATING

This coating is applied on lens surface to reduce adhesion of water and oil droplets. Thus, the lens can be cleaned easily. It is a special layer of silicone deposits.

POLAROID LENSES

These lenses remove glare reflected from flat surfaces like water, highways and snow. They protect against UV rays and improve visibility due to reduced glare. Polarizing material is nitrocellulose packed with ultramicroscopic crystals of herapathite. Transmittance of light through the lens is remarkably decreased. These lenses are available in glass, resin and polycarbonate materials (Chapter 1, Polarization of Light).

ULTRAVIOLET PROTECTIVE GLASSES

These lenses absorb UV rays and protect against their harmful effects. They are more suitable for persons who have to work outdoors for long hours. If exposed to UV rays, a person may develop snow blindness, pterygium and pinguecula. Ultraviolet rays are of three types: UV-A (200–280 nm), UV-B (280–315 nm) and UV-C (315–400 nm). Ozone layer in the earth's atmosphere absorbs UV-C rays from sunlight. Crown glass can absorb UV rays up to 300 nm and resin lenses can absorb UV rays up to 350 nm. Polycarbonate lenses can absorb all harmful UV rays. UV protective coating applied on resin lenses can also absorb all UV rays (up to 400 nm). UV coating imparts a very light yellow hue to the lens. These protective glasses also contain filters which block infrared rays harmful to human retina (Infrared A rays 700–1400 nm).

BALANCE LENS

This type of lens is used to balance the weight of the other lens in the spectacle frame where one eye is practically blind. For better cosmetic appearance, the balance lens power and style should match the other lens.

OPTICAL CENTER OF A LENS

It is a point in the lens from which rays of light pass undeviated. To understand the concept it is essential to know that a convex lens is made up of prisms placed base-to-base. Hence, the power is maximum at edges and zero in the center.

Clinical Significance

Clinical significance of optical center is that fitting of glasses in frame should be such that the optical center falls against the center of pupil so that there is no prismatic effect.

How to Find Optical Center of a Lens

It can be done with lensometer and manual method.

By Lensometer

Place a lens on the platform (lens holder) and look through eyepiece. Looking through the eyepiece moves the lens in such a way that the green circle (target of lensometer) should fall exactly on the center of the black cross. Mark the point with a marker. This is the optical center of the lens.

Manual Method

See a bright straight line like image of a tube light through lens. It appears double. Move the lens up down so that the two images superimpose upon each other. With a marker, mark this line on lens.

Repeat the procedure by rotating the lens by 90°. The point where two lines cross is the optical center of lens.

GHOST IMAGES

These are spurious images experienced by some persons usually low myopes. These are formed as a result of reflections of light from front as well as back surface of the lens and from the front surface of cornea. Complaints about ghost images are relatively rare. Most common offender is the reflection from back and front lens surfaces of a small light source in front of the patient in a dark area. Patient complains that he sees extra images of streetlights at night. The patient may also complain of seeing double. A careful history can diagnose the complaint, and counseling usually takes care of it. Streak reflections may be produced in bifocals by reflection off the segment tops. Patients perceive vertical streaks or bars of light **(Fig. 9.5)**.

Different techniques suggested for dealing with ghost image problems are:

- **Adjusting base curve or pantoscopic tilt:** This may move images slightly, but won't get rid of them. Adjustment is usually ineffective.
- **Decentration:** The idea here is to move ghost images, especially those formed by objects in front of the patient. It does not work.
- **Changing base curve:** It is completely irrelevant to images of objects in front of the patient and will make only a negligible difference for objects behind.

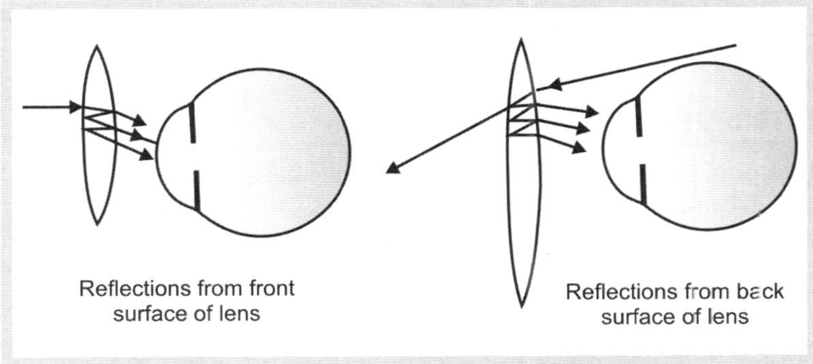

Fig. 9.5: Mechanism of ghost images.

- **Contact lenses:** This works perfectly optically, but may not be practical for some patients like patients who require low cylindrical lens.
- **Counseling:** This is the most common and best approach. Once patients understand the origin and inevitability of the ghost image problem, they can usually adapt.
- **Change bifocal style:** Changing to a fused bifocal or progressive will help with vertical streaks.
- **Antireflective coating:** The reduction of reflections with a single coating is incomplete but multiple layers can help further to reduce amplitude and to cancel out light at several wavelengths. As many as 9 layers may be used cancelling up to 99.5% of reflected light. Many of these coatings are protective as well. This is a practical and useful method.

TILTING OF LENSES

Spectacles should be worn in such a way that the lenses lie perpendicular to the visual axis. Thus, the incident light falls upon them normally, i.e., at an angle of 90°. If a lens is worn in a tilted manner, its spherical power is increased and cylindrical power is introduced. This change in power is not significant if power is low but in high-powered lenses this becomes very significant and can cause eye strain symptoms.

VERTEX DISTANCE

This is the distance in mm from back surface of spectacle lens to front surface of cornea. This is around 12 mm and should be kept same as change of this distance changes effectivity of lens. Anterior displacement of convex lens increases its effectivity and anterior displacement of concave lens decreases its effectivity (Chapter 3, Effectivity of Lens).

INTERPUPILLARY DISTANCE

Interpupillary distance (IPD) is the distance between center of pupil of one eye and center of pupil of another eye. This is very important for fitting of every type of spectacle lenses especially progressive addition lenses. This is to avoid any type of decentration of lenses and thus prismatic effect. Distance from center of pupil of one eye and midpoint of nasal bridge is known as monocular pupillary distance. This distance is of importance for PAL lenses as the face is often asymmetrical. IPD can be measured with a pupillometer and IPD ruler.

Measurement of IPD with IPD Ruler

Ask the patient to look into the left eye of examiner with his right eye. Place the zero point of ruler against center of pupil of patient's right eye. Now ask the patient to look into the right eye of examiner with his left eye and measure the distance in mm from pupil to pupil. Other ways of measuring IPD is from:

- Nasal pupil border of one eye to temporal pupil border of another eye in horizontal plane in cases of equal pupil size in both eyes.
- Nasal limbus of one eye to temporal limbus of another eye in horizontal plane in cases of anisocoria or lack of visibility of pupil.
- Nasal canthus of one eye to temporal canthus of other eye in case of uncooperative patients (but it is a less reliable method).
- IPD can also be measured with the help of a pupillometer.

Monocular Pupillary Distance

This is the distance taken in mm from center of pupil of one eye and center of nasal bridge keeping zero at the center of pupil.

Measurement of IPD with Pupillometer

The pupillometer uses corneal reflexes for measurements. It measures binocular as well as monocular PD, distance as well as near PD and PD at various distances like ∞, 60 cm, 50 cm, 40 cm. The advantages of pupillometer over manual IPD ruler is that it is easy to handle. It can be used by one-eyed practitioner or by the ones who have difficulty in closing one eye.

THE PRESCRIPTION

It should bear the following details:

Name of clinic/optical center

Name		*Age*		*Sex*	*Dated*			
		Right eye				*Left eye*		
	SPH	CYL	AXIS	VISION	SPH	CYL	AXIS	VISION
DIST.								
NEAR								

Type of lens-glass/CR/ARC/Photochromatic, etc.
Unifocal/Bifocal IPD
for constant use/near use

Name and signature of optometrist with regd. no

Common abbreviations used in clinical practice:

OD (Oculus dexter)—right eye (RE) OU (Oculi uterque)—both eyes (BE)	OS (Oculus sinister)—Left eye (LE) VR (Visus remotum)—For distance vision
VP (Visus Proximum)—For near vision NAD—No abnormality detected WNL—Within normal limits CST—Continue same treatment BU—Base-up Prism	Add—Near addition power- FU—Follow up
BO—Base-out prism OE—On examination ESO—Esophoria	IOP—Intraocular pressure BD—Base-down prism BI—Base in prism PMT—Post mydriatic test ET—Esotropia XT—Exotropia
EXO—Exophoria RH—Right hyperphoria RHT—Right hypertropia	LH—Left hyperphoria LHT—Left hypertropia

SPECIAL TYPES OF LENSES

High-index Lenses

Lenses with refractive index between 1.64 and 1.73 are called high index lenses. Lenses with refractive index more than this are called very high index lenses. These lenses are available in both glass and resin lenses.

Advantages of High-index Lenses

- Very thin and light weight
- Cosmetically better
- Better optics due to less aberration in high-power lenses
  More suitable for myopes because edge becomes very thin

However, transverse chromatic aberration is more and there is high surface reflectance. As a result the patient complains of colored tinge around the object when seen through high-index glasses.

Lenticular Lenses

These types of lenses are made when high-power lens is required. The purpose of making lenticular lens is to reduce its weight. The central portion of lens is called aperture, which gives dioptric power to the lens.

Lenticular lenses are of two types:
1. Minus/concave lenticular lenses
2. Plus/convex lenticular lenses

Aspheric Lenses

These types of lenses are made to neutralize spherical aberration by reducing the power of lens from center to periphery. Thus a +10DS aspheric lens will have +10D power in the center and +6D power at the periphery. This asphericity increases the field of vision with negligible prismatic effect. These lenses are available in glass, resin and high-index resin lens in the range of +6.00 DS to –15.00 DS. They are also available as single vision, bifocal and progressive addition lenses.

Protective Lenses

It is a special variety of lenses advised for children, sportspersons and industrial workers and all those professionals who are engaged in hazardous industries. These lenses are impact resistant and minimize the damage caused to eyeball in case of accidents. Such glasses can be made by:
- **Heat treatment:** A polished glass is melted and then cooled by cool air on both surfaces. Surface of the lens cools faster than the interior of the lens and brings surface of lens in a state of compression. Such lenses can be identified by the fact that they unpolarize the polarized light.
- Lamination of lenses makes them protective. If such a lens gets broken, there is little chance of injury to the eyeball.
- **Chemical treatment:** A finished lens is placed in a hot solution of potassium for 14 hours. Sodium ions are replaced by potassium ions. Now this lens is cooled which makes the surface of lens in a state of compression. It imparts impact resistance properties to the lens. Such lenses cannot unpolarize the polarized light.

Protective lenses may also be used to protect the eyes from radiations like photochromic lenses, lenses with antiglare coating, polaroid goggles, tinted lenses, UV absorbing lenses, etc.

10 CHAPTER

Spectacle Frames

FRAMES

A spectacle frame is a device used to hold the spectacle lenses in position and put them in front of eyes so that they can be used for seeing. A frame has broadly two parts: front and sides. Front part of a frame has joints, rim, bridge, pads and grooves. Eyewire, frame front or rim is that part of frame which holds lenses. Bridge is the middle part of the frame which joins two eyewires. Pads are synthetic parts which rest on nose. They are either screwed or snapped into the metal piece. Hinge is the part which joins sides with eyewires **(Fig. 10.1)**.

A side has again joints, thicker portion of the side called butt, bent portion of the side and sleeves. Certain terms which are commonly used with frames are:

- **Mount:** To fix the lenses in eyewire
- **Dismount:** To remove the lenses out of the eyewires
- **Temple length:** It is the length of side in mm.
- **Dowel point:** Point where hinge is located for connecting eyewire and temple.

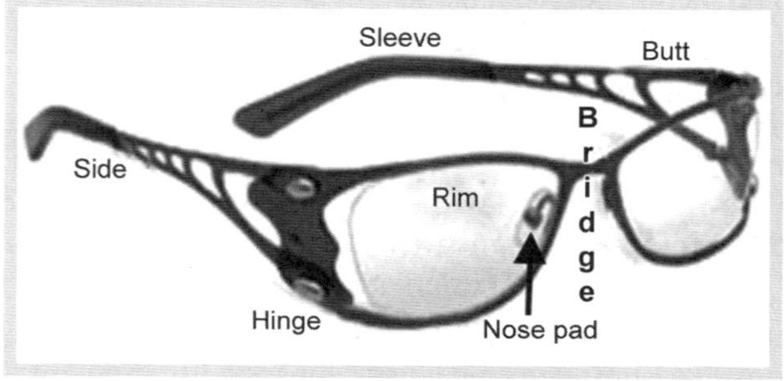

Fig. 10.1: Spectacle frame.

Lenticular Lenses

These types of lenses are made when high-power lens is required. The purpose of making lenticular lens is to reduce its weight. The central portion of lens is called aperture, which gives dioptric power to the lens.

Lenticular lenses are of two types:
1. Minus/concave lenticular lenses
2. Plus/convex lenticular lenses

Aspheric Lenses

These types of lenses are made to neutralize spherical aberration by reducing the power of lens from center to periphery. Thus a +10DS aspheric lens will have +10D power in the center and +6D power at the periphery. This asphericity increases the field of vision with negligible prismatic effect. These lenses are available in glass, resin and high-index resin lens in the range of +6.00 DS to –15.00 DS. They are also available as single vision, bifocal and progressive addition lenses.

Protective Lenses

It is a special variety of lenses advised for children, sportspersons and industrial workers and all those professionals who are engaged in hazardous industries. These lenses are impact resistant and minimize the damage caused to eyeball in case of accidents. Such glasses can be made by:

- **Heat treatment:** A polished glass is melted and then cooled by cool air on both surfaces. Surface of the lens cools faster than the interior of the lens and brings surface of lens in a state of compression. Such lenses can be identified by the fact that they unpolarize the polarized light.
- Lamination of lenses makes them protective. If such a lens gets broken, there is little chance of injury to the eyeball.
- **Chemical treatment:** A finished lens is placed in a hot solution of potassium for 14 hours. Sodium ions are replaced by potassium ions. Now this lens is cooled which makes the surface of lens in a state of compression. It imparts impact resistance properties to the lens. Such lenses cannot unpolarize the polarized light.

Protective lenses may also be used to protect the eyes from radiations like photochromic lenses, lenses with antiglare coating, polaroid goggles, tinted lenses, UV absorbing lenses, etc.

10
CHAPTER

Spectacle Frames

FRAMES

A spectacle frame is a device used to hold the spectacle lenses in position and put them in front of eyes so that they can be used for seeing. A frame has broadly two parts: front and sides. Front part of a frame has joints, rim, bridge, pads and grooves. Eyewire, frame front or rim is that part of frame which holds lenses. Bridge is the middle part of the frame which joins two eyewires. Pads are synthetic parts which rest on nose. They are either screwed or snapped into the metal piece. Hinge is the part which joins sides with eyewires **(Fig. 10.1)**.

A side has again joints, thicker portion of the side called butt, bent portion of the side and sleeves. Certain terms which are commonly used with frames are:

- **Mount:** To fix the lenses in eyewire
- **Dismount:** To remove the lenses out of the eyewires
- **Temple length:** It is the length of side in mm.
- **Dowel point:** Point where hinge is located for connecting eyewire and temple.

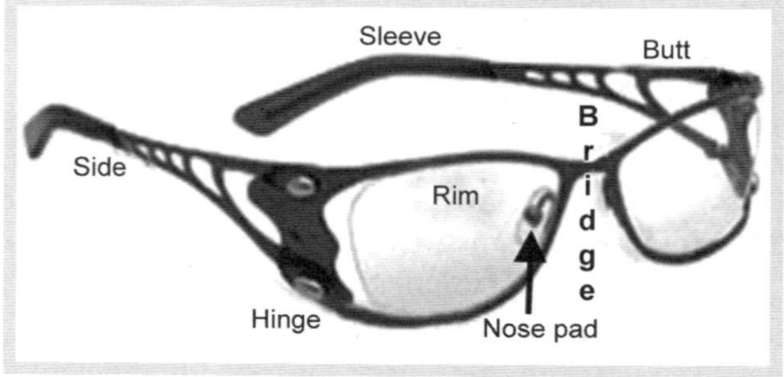

Fig. 10.1: Spectacle frame.

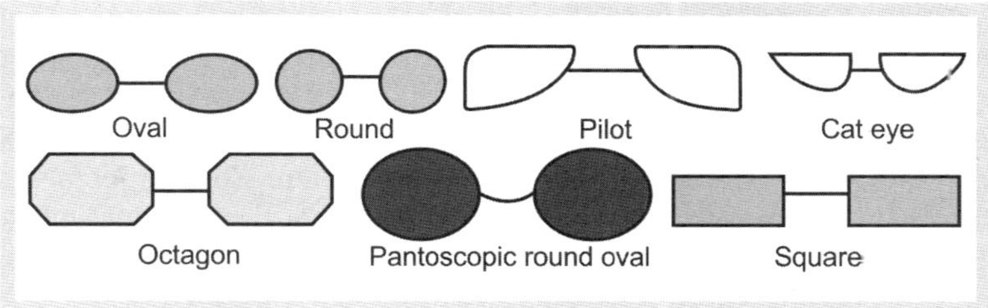

Fig. 10.2: Shapes of frames.

Shapes of Frames

Commonly used frames are of the following shapes **(Fig. 10.2)**:

- Square
- Oval
- Octagon
- Pilot or aviator
- Cat eye
- Round
- Pantoscopic round oval

Types of Frames

Full Rim

Lens is held in position by a metallic or some other material like plastic all around.

Half Rim or Supra

Here a metallic rim on one side and a fine nylon cord on other side hold the lenses in position. Nylon cord is attached to the rim. Rim may be on upper side or lower side. Consequently, the nylon cord is on the lower or upper side. Sometimes the rim may surround the lens all around but on lateral sides where there is nylon cord holding the lenses.

Rimless or Drill Mount

Here there is no rim around the lenses and the lenses are held in position by screws to the bridge and the temples. This is also known as three-piece frame because it has a nose bridge and two temples. Screws are fitted at four places, two temporal and two nasals

There are certain special types of spectacles like half eye. This is a small-sized spectacle used for reading purposes so that distant object can be seen over top of the spectacles. Certain sports variety goggles are also available like swimming goggles, squash goggles, divers goggles, snooker goggles, ski goggles, etc. Some spectacles are used for some specific occupation like welding spectacles, ptosis spectacles, low-vision aid spectacles, hearing aid spectacles, etc.

Clip-ons

These are also known as clip-on sunglasses or clip-on-glasses or clipon frames. These are detachable frames which can be used over regular glasses so that the wearer gets benefit of both prescription glasses and sun protection. Usually, they are tinted lenses or sunglasses.

Parts of a Frame

- **Bridge:** Area of frame which rests on the nose.
- **Rim/eyewire:** This part of the frame surrounds the lenses.
- **Endpieces/hinge:** These connect the front of the frame to the temple.
- **Nose pads:** Plastic pieces that rest on the nose which can sometimes be attached with metal guard arms.
- **Temple:** Part of the frame which follows the temple area and rests behind the ear. It is further divided into portions called butt portion (portion nearest to frame front), bend (where it bends over the ear), shank/shaft (portion between butt and bend).

Information Available from a Frame

Following type of information is always available from a frame **(Fig. 10.3)**.

- **Size of rim:** Length and width of rim is inscribed on the demo lenses in mm. It is technically called the horizontal boxed lens size. It can also be seen on the inner side of temple.
- **Temple length:** It is inscribed on the inner side of temple in mm.
- **Bridge size:** It is also called distance between lenses (DBL). It is inscribed on the inner side of temple.
- **Model number:** Name of manufacturer and color code of the frame is also inscribed on the inner side of temple.

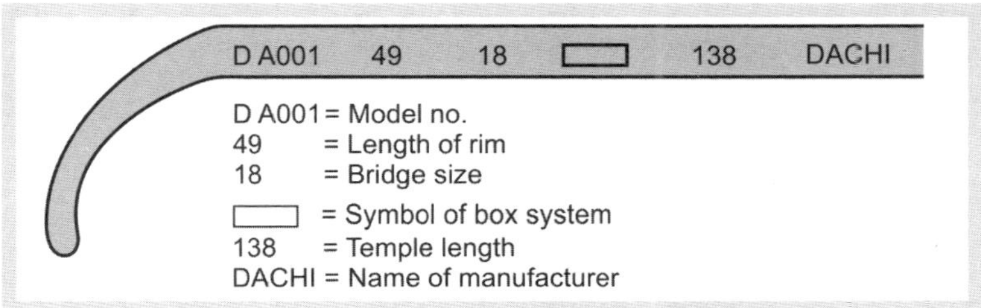

Fig. 10.3: Information available from a frame.

Selection of a Frame

A good frame should be comfortable. It should sit properly on the nose and behind the ears. It should be suitable for lenses to be fitted. High power lenses are thicker and heavy, hence the frame should be thicker to hold the lens. If the lenses are bifocal, the frames should be wide enough to fit both distance and near powers. It should be of the proper size, i.e., neither too big, too small nor too heavy. It must suit the face. The color of frame should complement skin and age.

A suitable spectacle frame adds charm to one's personality so one should wear frames according to their face shapes:

- **Round face:** A narrow frame with high set temples lengthens face.
- **Oval face:** It looks good in most styles.
- **Long face:** A larger square frame gives balance to a long face.
- **Pear-shaped with narrow forehead:** Frames with a strong top bar add width to forehead.
- **Long nose:** A low-set bridge tries to shorten it.
- **Short nose:** Choose a high-set bridge.
- **Close-set eyes:** A thin and clear bridge adds width between them.
- **Wide-set eyes:** A colored bridge makes eyes appear closer.

BOX SYSTEM

This is a new internationally accepted system of frame dimensions. This has replaced the previous Datum System. Different terms used in spectacle frames are **(Fig. 10.4)**:

- **Horizontal center line:** It is a horizontal line passing through the geometrical centers of two rims.
- **Vertical center line:** It is a vertical line passing through the geometrical centers of two rims.

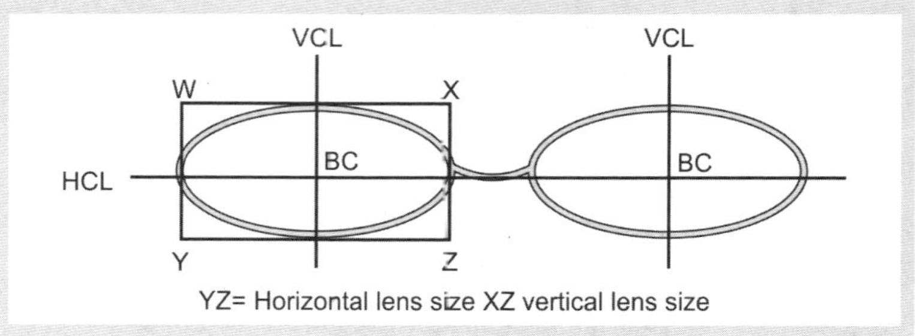

Fig. 10.4: Box system.

- **Horizontal lens size/A size:** It is the distance in mm between two vertical sides of rim.
- **Vertical lens size/B size:** It is the distance in mm between two horizontal sides of rim.
- **Boxed center/geometric center:** It is the point of intersection of horizontal and vertical center lines.
- **Distance between the lenses measurement (DBL):** It is the bridge size. It is measured from the inside nasal point of one to the inside nasal point of the other rim.
- **Distance between the rims measurement (DBR):** It is the distance between the rims at a specified level.
- **Effective diameter:** It is double the distance from pupillary center of the lens to the apex of lens bevel farthest from it. This measurement is mandatory for PALs fitting.
- **Segment height:** The difference between the top of the segment to the lower line of the boxing system rectangle enclosing the lens shape.

SPECTACLE FRAME MATERIALS

A variety of materials are available for making frames. An ideal spectacle frame material should have the following properties:

- It should be rigid enough.
- It should be flexible enough to give it different shapes.
- It should be economical.
- It should be long-lasting.
- It should be resistant to corrosion from sweat.
- It should be easily convertible into different shapes.
- It should be cosmetically attractive and soothing.

- It should be lightweight.
- It should not cause any allergic reaction to tissues it comes in contact with.

Metal frames usually consist of a number of different materials: the structural metal of the frame called the base metal and the plating material, frequently an organic lacquer (coating), and the plastic side tips and nose pads. Before coating, the wire is drawn through rollers to change it to the desired configuration. This hardens most alloys. Joints between the components of metal frames can either be made by soldering or by welding. Both soldering and welding weaken the heated area. Many alloys cannot be soldered or welded satisfactorily with the simple brazing torches used in practice. This is because an oxide layer forms very rapidly and prevents adhesion. Many metals are toxic and great care should be taken not to inhale any dust from these alloys. Even safe metals such as titanium and aluminum can be dangerous if the particle size is such as to cause lung damage.

Following types of materials are available for manufacturing of spectacle frames:

- **Stainless steel:** This is a durable material with flexibility. Spring effect can be given in the frame. It is suitable for patients who are prone to develop allergic reactions from ordinary frames. It needs to be electroplated or painted to prevent corrosion.
- **Aluminum:** It is very economic, lightweight, cosmetically attractive and resistant to corrosion. It is a soft material, so sides are made thick. It is possible to add decorative finish to the material. It is a very good conductor of heat hence becomes very cold in winters and hot in summers. So the temple (two long sides) needs to be covered with plastic sleeves. There are fewer chances of allergic reactions from this material.
- **German silver:** It is corrosion resistant and flexible but needs electroplating with nickel and is quite allergenic hence can cause allergic reactions in susceptible individuals.
- **Titanium:** It is most lightweight of all frames, 40% lighter than normal frame materials, highly corrosion resistant from sweat, heat resistant and nonallergic. Different colors can be added in it to make it more attractive. But they are very costly. It has very good memory, i.e., it retains its original configuration. It is available as pure titanium, clad titanium and a combination of both.

- **Rolled gold:** This is a precious metal frame. The process by which these frames are made makes the product become harder and springier. This metal occupies the upper end of the gold frame market.
- **9 carat gold** is also used to make frames. It is very resistant to corrosion, easily adjustable and convenient to work with.
- **Nickel silver:** This is 12–25% nickel but mostly copper. It is mechanically quite a good material for spectacle frames, but it becomes dull very quickly if not plated or coated and rapidly turns green in contact with body fluids. It is easily worked and soldered and is one of the most common materials for spectacle frames. Nickel silver is commonly used for the joints and side reinforcement of plastic frames. Allergy to nickel and its alloys is common but it only presents a problem where the metal is in contact with the skin. However, this can be prevented by using plastic side-tips and bridges of inert metal or polymer coatings.
- **Memory metals:** This is a group of alloys which has the common property of being able to return to their original shape after considerable distortion. They do snap if repeatedly flexed through sharp angles. Frames are seldom made from memory metals alone. These materials are commonly used for temples and bridges with more conventional materials used for the eyewire screws and other parts. This is because of cost factor and they are so flexible that they cannot be adjusted satisfactorily. The best known memory metal is nickel, titanium but it is often sold as a titanium alloy with no mention of nickel. There are also other memory effect metals like aluminum, titanium-cobalt and aluminium-vanadium-titanium, etc.
- **Combination of materials:** Sometimes one part of a frame is made from one material and the other part is made from a different material, for example metals and plastics. This does not include a plastic front with metal joints, or a metal front with plastic nose pads. It also does not include composites. In practice, almost all frames are made from combinations of materials—plastic fronts commonly have metal sides and vice versa. Similarly, plastic sides usually have metal reinforcement while metal sides usually have plastic tips.
- **Plastics:** Hawksbill turtle, the source of natural plastic, has been declared endangered species by the World Wildlife Fund. Hence

natural plastics like turtle shell, bone, horn, ivory, leather and wood have become obsolete nowadays. Synthetic plastic is of two types: thermoplastics and thermosetting. Thermoplastics can be reformed with heat and thermosetting cannot be reformed with heat because the material breaks up on exposure to heat. Plastic frames can be made from different materials like cellulose acetate, cellulose nitrate, cellulose propionate, cellulose acetate butyrate, PMMA, epoxy resins, polyamides (nylons), polycarbonate, silicone rubbers, carbon fiber, Kevlar and composite materials.

- **Cellulose acetate:** This is one of the best materials available and probably the most common plastic spectacle frame material. It is very light, strong, and mechanically stable at normal temperatures, easily worked and relatively inert. It is cosmetically attractive and a very transparent material. It tends to whiten where in contact with patient's body fluids particularly at the bridge and temples. It is attacked by some common solvents and dissolves in acetone. Acetate sides usually have full-length wire reinforcement and any color is usually throughout the material. It softens at around 50°C temperature so prone to damage by excess heat.
- **Cellulose nitrate:** Cellulose nitrate is very similar to cellulose acetate but it catches fire at a temperature little above required to adjust it. It is strong, convenient to work with and its surface can be polished brightly. It becomes dark "urine-yellow" color and very brittle with age.
- **Polyamides (nylons):** These are very rarely called "Nylons". The materials are used in sunglasses, sports spectacles, safety spectacles and temporary aphakic spectacles. They are very strong, but have a very soft surface, can be very flexible and often cannot be adjusted with ordinary frame heaters.
- **Carbon fiber graphite:** It is very light, heat resistant, durable and strong. It is one of the favored materials for manufacturers of frames.
- **Polycarbonate:** This is best known as a lens material and is very strong. Its use as a frame material is uncommon, other than for sports and saftey spectacles.
- **Silicone rubbers:** These are soft, flexible materials, used for bridges, side-tips, rim-liners, etc. They are extremely stable and typically retain their elastic properties from –50 to 200°C.

- **Cellulose acetate butyrate (CAB):** It is occasionally used for safety spectacles. Little information is available on its properties as a spectacle frame material. Some of the plastic side tips of metal frames may be made from it.
- **Polymethyl methacrylate/acrylic resins:** This is remarkably transparent, cosmetically good looking, highly stable but has low resistance to impact and not convenient to work with as it is very brittle. This is almost obsolete as a frame material.
- **Epoxy/epoxide resins:** Epoxy frames are usually translucent, but opaque colors have also been available (in this case the body of the material is usually white, and is again colored with a surface dye). These frames have been claimed to be hypoallergenic. They are usually coated with a transparent lacquer both to protect them and reduce their allergenic potential.
- **Kevlar:** This is another material now in occasional use. It is what "bullet-proof vests" are made from.

Headache after Using Spectacles: How to Manage?

INTRODUCTION

This is not a very infrequent complaint. A patient is prescribed glasses and sent home satisfactorily but a day or two he comes with a complaint of headache. This is how one can proceed to pinpoint the diagnosis.

Something to be Done on the Part of Optometrist/Ophthalmologist

- Incorrect prescription—even slight error of power especially cylindrical or wrong axis of glass may cause headache. Due care must be taken while prescribing the power to any patient especially those who are involved in reading, writing, watching TV for long hours or working on computer.
- If refractive error has been over or under corrected, rectification in prescription should be done accordingly.

Something to be Done on the Part of Optician

- Power of spectacles does not match the power prescribed—change the glasses as per prescription.
- Even change in size of glasses sometimes makes the patient uncomfortable. Patient should be explained about the cause and frame may be selected accordingly.
- If the glasses are not centered properly they cause discomfort. Proper centering should be done.
- Tilting of lenses introduces cylindrical power and changes effective power of lens, which becomes a source of trouble. Patient should be advised to wear spectacles properly.
- If patient complains of glare, prescribe antiglare glasses.

Something to be Done on the Part of Patient Himself

- If power of glasses is high like in aphakia or high myopia, there is peripheral distortion of image. Patient should be advised to look through center of glass and not through periphery of glass.
- If best-corrected vision is less than required by patient, e.g., due to ARMD or anisometropia or amblyopia, patient might have some problem in doing near work for long hours.
- A beginner takes time to adjust with bifocal and multifocal (progressive) glasses. He should be advised to wait for some time and try to adjust with the glasses. However, some patients cannot adjust in spite of all efforts. It is better for them to use separate pair of glasses for distance and near.
- Some patients take time to adjust with new pair of spectacles, so if a person is well adjusted with previous glasses and there is not much change in power, advise him to continue with same glass.
- Sudden change in power causes trouble. Give time for adjustment.
- Hypermetropes usually take time to adjust with glasses, so wait and watch for some time.
- If spectacles are worn in a wrong fashion, i.e., back vertex distance is changed, e.g., too low or too high on nose, it causes trouble. Patient should be advised to wear glasses properly.
- Patient is having exophoria and needs muscle exercises. Such patients usually complain of headache while doing near work. Convergence exercises should be advised.
- Contrast sensitivity of patient is decreased due to cataract or glaucoma, so he is not satisfied due to fogginess of vision. He should be explained about the nature of disease and all efforts should be made to treat the underlying cause.
- Patient does not like glasses or is not in a habit of using glasses. He should be explained the advantages of using glasses and should be encouraged to use glasses.

CHAPTER 12 Ophthalmic Procedures and Instruments

LENS AND LOUPE

This is a very handy instrument used to examine structures of anterior segment of eyeball. It consists of a condensing lens of +13D and a corneal loupe of power +41D (consisting of two plano-convex lenses of power +20.5D each) with 10 × magnification. It is based on the *principle* that when an object is placed between a convex lens and its focus, the image formed is erect, magnified, virtual and on the same side of the lens **(Figs. 12.1 and 12.2)**.

Technique

Patient is seated on a stool with a light source coming from front and lateral side from a distance of two feet. Condensing lens is held in one hand and used to focus light on structure to be examined. Loupe is held in other hand between thumb and index finger. Little finger and ring fingers are rested on forehead for stability of hand and upper eyelid is lifted with middle finger. Loupe is brought close to the eye so that the cornea comes into focus. By changing the position of condensing lens, corneal loupe and position of eyes of observer; different structures of anterior segment can be examined one by one.

Lens and Loupe has fallen into disrepute with more and more use of *binocular loupe* and slit lamp. Binocular loupe has the added advantage of binocularity but magnification is lesser as compared to uniocular loupe. It is fixed to the examiner's head hence lesser maneuver is required.

SLIT LAMP

Uses

- It is used for detailed examination of anterior segment. It gives a stereoscopic and magnified view of the part examined.

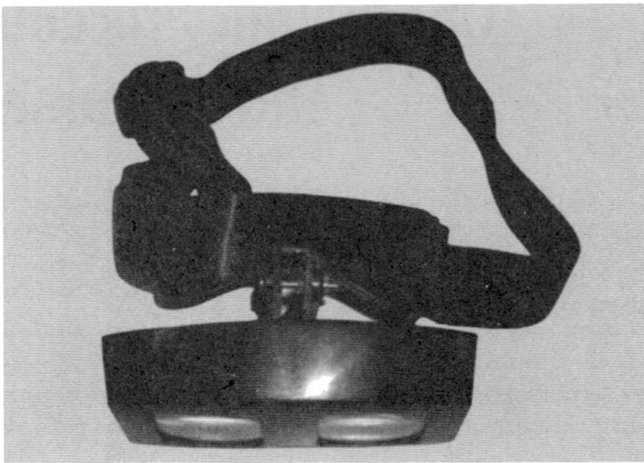

Fig. 12.1: Binocular loupe.

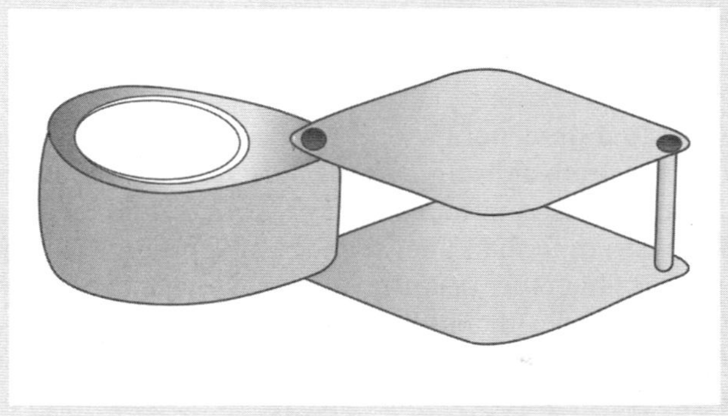

Fig. 12.2: Corneal loupe.

- It is required for examination of angle of anterior chamber with gonioscope.
- Measurement of IOP with applanation tonometer requires slit lamp.
- Delivery of laser like YAG, argon and diode can be done only through slit lamp.
- It is used for detailed examination of retina by slit lamp biomicroscopy.
- Vital staining of cornea is observed through slit lamp.

Parts of Slit Lamp

Slit lamp can be divided into two main parts **(Fig. 12.3)**:

1. Illumination system
2. Observation system

Illumination system consists of a light source that can be moved away from observation system so that a particular angle can be made between illumination system and the observation system. This is required for different techniques of slit lamp examination.

Intensity of light source can be increased or decreased as per requirement by rotating a knob or rheostat. Another knob can change the height and diameter of light beam. Width of light beam can also be changed via another knob.

Halogen light is used in most of the examinations. Different filters like cobalt blue filter are used for fluoresein staining, fitting of rigid gas permeable contact lens and applanation tonometer. Red free (green) filter is used for seeing nerve fiber bundle defects in glaucoma. Blood vessels, microaneurysms and hemorrhages appear dark against a green background with a red free filter. Vitreous details are also seen better with blue or green light as they have shorter wavelengths and have more scattering properties. Yellow filter improves contrast as scattering of blue light is no more there. All these filters can be introduced using a knob.

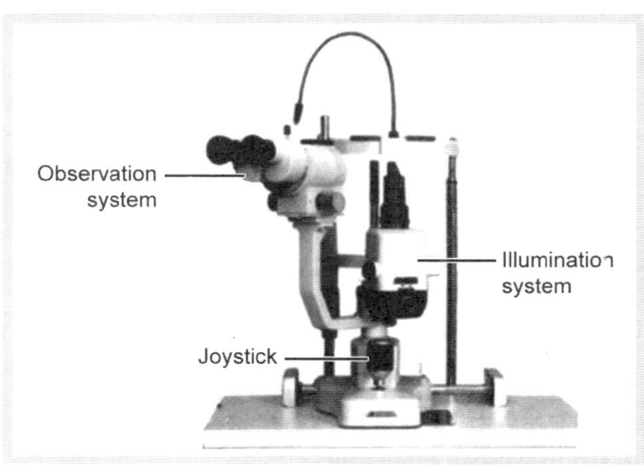

Fig. 12.3: Slit lamp.

Observation system consists of two eyepieces. Magnification of image is obtained by multiplying the power of oculars with the power of the objective lens. Magnification can be changed either by changing the objective lens or the oculars. This is achieved by flipping a lever located below the observation system.

Focusing is controlled by a joystick. It is designed to move the slit lamp laterally and forwards and backwards. Vertical movement is done by rotating the joystick.

Techniques of Slit-lamp Examination

1. Diffuse illumination
2. Direct illumination
3. Indirect illumination
4. Retro illumination

Diffuse Illumination

It is used to examine different structures of eyeball like eyelids, cornea, conjunctiva, sclera, iris, pupil, etc. It gives general information. A frosted glass or ground glass is placed in front of the focused light beam to get diffuse illumination. Magnification is kept low and incident light is projected into the eyeball obliquely at an angle of 45°.

Direct Illumination

Viewing of structures within the focused light beam is known as direct illumination. It may be of different types:

- **Optical section:** Light beam is in form of a slit. It is projected obliquely. The angle between the oculars and observation system is 30–60°. More is the angle, wider is the optical section called parallelepiped. It gives a cross sectional view of different layers of cornea. Lens and anterior part of vitreous can also be examined in a dilated pupil. This technique is applied to locate corneal lesion, corneal scar, foreign body, depth of AC and type of cataract.
- **Conical/pinpoint illumination:** This technique is used to look for aqueous flare and cells in AC in uveitis. The room should be absolutely dark. Beam is pin point and focused against pupil in the AC. Aqueous flare appears as yellowish particles and cells in AC appear as whitish reflections.

- **Specular reflection:** It is used to see corneal endothelium. It is best seen with one eyepiece only. Angle of illumination system is set equal to the angle of the oculars and illumination beam is a parallelepiped. First of all corneal surface is focused with low magnification. Move the oculars 20–30° away from illumination source. Now move the illumination source 20–30° away and in opposite direction until a bright mirror like reflection is seen through one ocular. Three reflections are seen. Intermediate reflection is focused finely using high magnification and endothelial cells can be counted.

Indirect Illumination

Here structures not within the focused light beam but adjacent to the focused light beam are observed. It is of different types:

- **Proximal illumination:** A moderately wide beam of light is focused on the areas adjacent to the areas of interest. The lesion is observed with scattered light against dark background.
- **Sclerotic scatter:** Lesions within the corneal substance can be seen by this method. A parallelepiped illumination beam is focused at the temporal limbus. Eyepiece is focused on central part of cornea and illumination system is set at an angle between 45 to 60° with the observation system. Light beam enters corneal substance from one limbus, undergoes total internal reflection and exits from opposite limbus.

Retro Illumination

In this technique light is reflected from iris or retina to see more anteriorly located structures. It may be of different types:

- In *direct retro illumination* light is focused behind the structure to be seen and it is angled at 45°. Corneal opacity appears black against illuminated background. Lenticular opacities appear dark against red glow of fundus. Thus objects that normally appear bright are seen as black in this technique.
- In *indirect retro illumination* light is focused in such a way that the background becomes dark. The structure to be seen should not be in the pathway of light.

There is another technique called *transillumination*. In this technique iris surface is tested for passage of light. Illumination system and observation system are positioned coaxially, i.e., click stop position. Red glow seen through iris confirms hole in the iris.

TONOMETRY

It is a procedure by which we measure the intraocular pressure of eyeball. The instrument used is known as tonometer. Normal IOP of human eyeball is between 10 and 20 mm Hg. If it is more than normal; it damages retina and optic nerve and makes the patient blind. This condition is known as glaucoma.

Types

It is of two types:

1. **Digital tonometry:** By this method, we palpate the eyeball with pulp of fingers and assess how soft or hard it is. The readings are noted as stony hard (very high IOP), hard (high IOP) or soft (normal IOP). This gives us reasonably reliable information but cannot tell precisely the IOP. However, it can be done at any time and on every patient. There is no instrumentation required.
2. **Instrumental tonometry:** It is done by using an instrument. This measures IOP more precisely. It is of two types:
   i. **Applanation tonometry:** It is the best method to measure IOP. However, it requires costly equipments like slit lamp and applanation tonometer **(Fig. 12.4A)** and requires more expertise, e.g., Goldmann applanation tonometer, noncontact tonometer.
   ii. **Indentation (impression) tonometry:** This is the most commonly employed method of measuring IOP. The principle states that the degree of indentation is proportional to IOP. This requires only tonometer which is very handy and economical, e.g., Schiotz tonometer **(Fig. 12.4B)**. It measures the depth of impression produced by a small plunger carrying a known weight. The IOP is determined by correlating scale reading using a nomogram.

Procedure of Schiotz Tonometry

Make the patient lie down comfortably in bed. Put a drop of local anesthetic agent like lignocaine or proparacaine. Take a clean and sterilized tonometer. Ask the patient to fix his eyes on his thumb or roof such that they are exactly at right angle to the earth. Place the tonometer on his cornea and record the reading on scale. Repeat the procedure in other eye. Convert this scale reading into IOP by seeing conversion table. This gives the IOP **(Fig. 12.5)**.

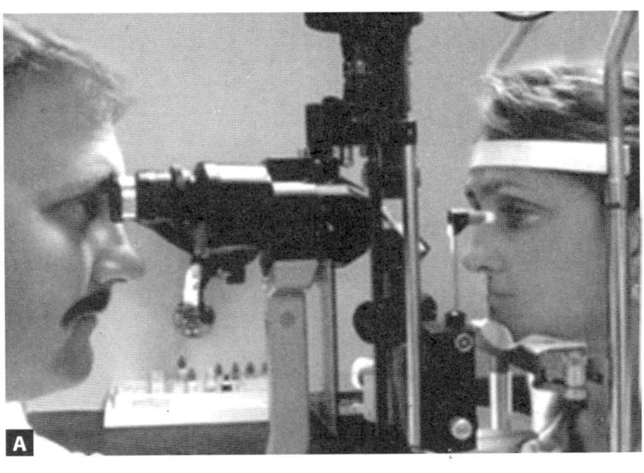

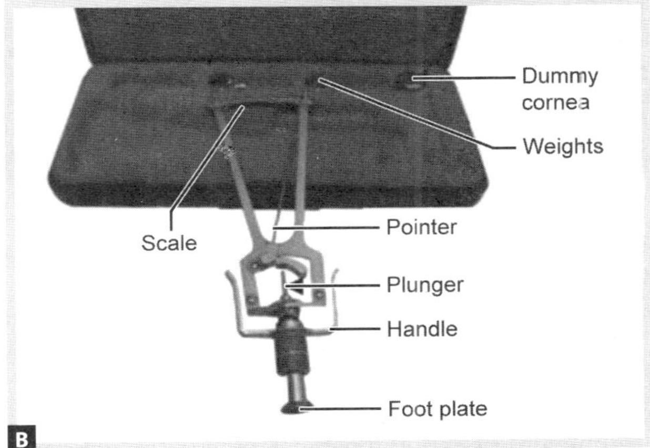

Figs. 12.4A and B: (A) Applanation tonometer; (B) Schiotz tonometer.

Normal weight of Schiotz tonometer is 5.5 g. It can be made 7.5 g, 10 g and 15 g by addition of weight provided with the instrument. If scale reading is less than three add weight and repeat the procedure. This increases the accuracy of the tonometer.

Advantages of Schiotz Tonometer

Very simple procedure, easy to do, economical and handy instrumentation is required.

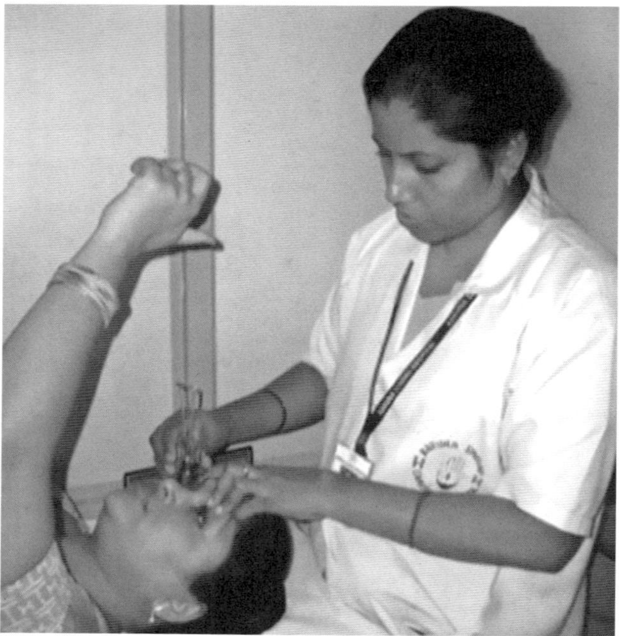

Fig. 12.5: Procedure of Schiotz tonometry.

Disadvantages of Schiotz Tonometer

It can introduce infection in the eyeball. To prevent it, tonometer should be sterilized prior to use and antibiotic should be instilled in the eye after the procedure. If patient moves the eyeball during the procedure; cornea may be injured. To prevent this complication the procedure and risk should be explained to the patient properly and proper anesthesia should be achieved before carrying out the procedure.

Goldmann applanation tonometry is considered the most reliable and best method to measure IOP. It works on the principle of Imbert Fick's law, i.e., pressure inside a sphere (P) is equal to force required to flatten a surface (F) divided by area of flattening.

$$P = F/A$$

It consists of a spring loaded lever and a biprism that are mounted on a slit-lamp. The area of cornea applanated by biprism is 3.06 mm.

Procedure of Goldmann applanation tonometer: The patient's eye is anesthetized with proparacaine (0.5%) followed by staining the tear film with fluorescein. Patient is seated in front of the slit lamp and cobalt blue filter is used to illuminate the cornea and biprism. The dial is set at 10 mm Hg. The biprism is slowly advanced toward the cornea. When the biprism just touches the cornea, the two semicircles are observed uniocularly from the slit lamp. Move the dial to the point such that the inner edges of the semicircles just touch each other. The readings are noted.

Sources of error: The common sources of error are highly toric corneas, lid touching the probe, improper cleaning of biprism, improper calibration, repeated readings of IOP and observer bias.

Perkin's tonometer is useful in children and patients under general anesthesia and those who cannot cooperate on slit lamp.

Noncontact tonometer (Fig. 12.6) or air puff tonometer uses rapid air pulse to applanate the cornea. An electro-optical system detects the corneal applanation. Force of air jet required to applanate the cornea determines the IOP. This is a very quick method and has no risk of infection as there is no touch with cornea. However it does not give accurate readings hence it is suitable only for screening purposes.

Sterilization of Schiotz Tonometer

It can be done by different methods:

- **Dry heat:** Foot plate of tonometer should be heated over flame for 10 seconds, cooled and reused. Repeated heating however, will distort the shape of foot plate and create erroneous readings.
- Use of ultraviolet rays
- Use of tonofilms
- Soak the assembled foot plate in a solution of 1:1000 merthiolate solution
- Clean the foot plate with a swab soaked with ethyl alcohol. This is the most common method employed clinically.

It is recommended that after each use the tonometer should be disassembled, barrel should be cleaned with a white pipe soaked with alcohol followed by another pipe which is dry. The foot plate, plunger and dummy cornea should be cleaned with swab soaked with alcohol and allowed to get dry for 60 seconds. Now it is ready to be placed on another cornea.

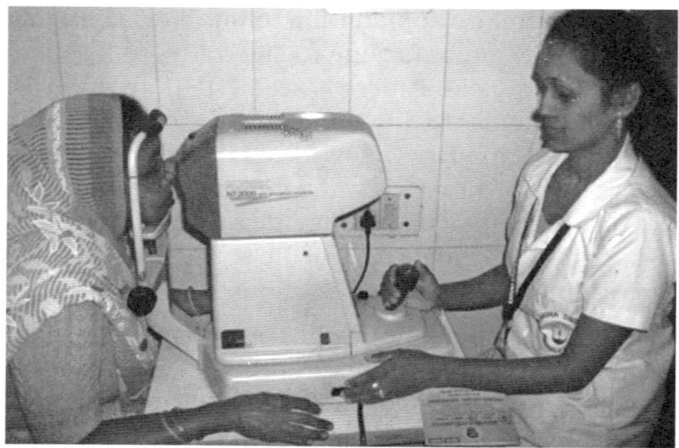

Fig. 12.6: Noncontact tonometry.

EPILATION AND ELECTROEPILATION

Due to certain causes like trachoma, injury and chemical burn eyelashes become misdirected and rub against cornea. This disturbs transparency of cornea and ultimately results in corneal blindness. To prevent it misdirected, eyelashes are removed under slit-lamp examination. The process of removing misdirected cilia is known as epilation. It is repeated every month because the removed cilia regrow.

If a small galvanic current is passed through follicle of eyelash, the follicle gets damaged and eyelash can be pulled easily. This process of removing misdirected cilia by passing galvanic current is known as electroepilation. Because the hair follicle gets damaged, so cilia do not regrow.

LACRIMAL SYRINGING

This is a procedure by which we check patency of lacrimal apparatus. Sometimes, it is done as a diagnostic as well as curative procedure.

Indications

- If patient complains of watering from one or both eyes and we suspect some abnormality of lacrimal drainage system, e.g., congenital dacryocystitis, chronic dacryocystitis, etc.

Conversion Table for Schiotz Tonometry

Scale reading	*5.5 g weight*	*7.5 g weight*	*10 g weight*	*15 g weight*
0.0	41.5	59.1	81.7	127.5
0.5	37.8	54.2	75.1	117.9
1.0	34.5	49.8	69.3	109.3
1.5	31.6	45.8	64.0	101.4
2.0	29	42.5	59.1	94.3
2.5	26.6	38.3	54.7	38.0
3.0	24.4	35.8	50.6	31.8
3.5	22.4	33.0	46.9	76.2
4.0	20.6	30.4	43.4	71.0
4.5	18.9	28.0	40.2	66.2
5.0	17.3	25.8	37.2	61.8
5.5	15.9	23.8	34.4	57.6
6.0	14.6	21.9	31.8	53.6
6.5	13.4	20.1	29.4	49.9
7.0	12.2	18.5	27.2	46.5
7.5	11.2	17.0	25.1	43.2
8.0	10.2	15.6	23.1	40.2
8.5	9.4	14.3	21.3	38.1
9.0	8.5	13.1	19.6	34.6
9.5	7.8	12.0	18.0	32.0
10.0	7.1	10.9	16.5	29.6

- After dacryocystorhinostomy (DCR) surgery; to check outcome of surgery.

Clinically regurgitation test also known as regurgitation on pressure over lacrimal sac (ROPLAS) test should be done prior to syringing. It gives very useful information. It is done by pressing the medial canthus with finger tip. Regurgitation of discharge confirms blockage of nasolacrimal duct.

Technique

Examine the patient under slit lamp and rule out agenesis of lacrimal punctum and punctual atresia. If puncta are normal; make the patient lie down on an examination table. Put one drop of local anesthetic agent like lignocaine or proparacaine. Take a 2 mL syringe with lacrimal cannula and fill it with normal saline. Introduce cannula into the punctum after dilating it with punctum dilator. Push saline slowly. Ask the patient if he feels presence of water in his mouth. If he says 'yes'; it means lacrimal drainage system is patent. Saline will come out of the same or opposite punctum if there is any blockage in the pathway.

Observations

- Fluid comes out through opposite punctum after initial delay. Site of blockage is nasolacrimal duct.
- Fluid comes out of opposite punctum immediately. Site of blockage is common canaliculus.
- Fluid comes out of same (lower or upper) punctum. Site of blockage is lower canaliculus or upper canaliculus.

To know the exact site of blockage another procedure is done known as *dacryocystography*. In this procedure Conray 280 dye is used instead of saline and after doing syringing a radiograph of eye portion is taken. The level of dye shows the exact site of blockage.

Complications

- Injury to the lacrimal punctum or canaliculus can occur.
- Creation of false passage.

FLUORESCEIN STAINING

It is a procedure by which we can stain and visualize all types of micro or macroabrasions of cornea easily. The name of the stain/dye is sodium fluorescein. It is available as 10% (5 mL) and 20% (3 mL) solution in form of ampoules or strips impregnated with the stain. This dye has an inherent property of fluorescence, i.e., it absorbs light of one wavelength (blue) and emits light of another wavelength (green). That is why the stained area appears green when seen through blue light.

Procedure

Put one drop of fluorescein dye in the eye or put the strip in lower conjunctival fornix for a few seconds. Ask the patient to blink eyes so that the stain spreads in the eyeball and then keep the eyes closed for 30 seconds. Wash excess of dye with normal saline and examine under slit lamp with cobalt blue filter. The stained area of cornea will appear green.

Uses

- We can easily visualize small injuries of cornea.
- Fluorescein dye is also used in some other tests like fluorescein dye disappearance test, Jones test to check function of lacrimal sac and fundus fluorescein angiography.

High molecular weight fluorescein is used for evaluation of fitting of contact lenses, e.g., piggy back lenses, hybrid lenses as it is not absorbed by the contact lens material.

CORNEAL SCRAPING

It is done in cases of corneal ulcer or corneal abscess. This procedure is carried out either under slit lamp or microscope. One drop of local anesthetic drug like paracaine is put in the eye, wait for 30 seconds so that local anesthesia is achieved. With the help of a hypodermic needle cornea is scraped and dead tissue is removed and sent for culture and sensitivity examination. This procedure should be carried out very gently to avoid corneal perforation.

Advantages of Scraping

- It removes dead tissue thus drug can penetrate the cornea better that helps in healing.
- Along with the dead tissue, the debris is also removed which contains pathogens. Thus the load of bacteria is also reduced.

CAUTERIZATION OF ULCERS

It is done for better healing of corneal ulcers. After scraping cornea is washed with normal saline. 1:5 diluted betadine lotion is applied over the ulcerated area. Carbolic acid (phenol) is applied over the margins of corneal ulcer. One drop of atropine is put in the eye. Pad and bandage is done with antibiotic eye ointment. This is known as chemical cauterization. It prevents extension of ulcer.

Instead of carbolic acid heat cautery can also be applied at the margins of the ulcer.

ESTHESIOMETRY

This is a procedure by which we check the corneal sensitivity. Sensitivity of cornea is decreased markedly in viral corneal ulcers, neuroparalytic keratitis. It is decreased to some extent in all types of affections of cornea. So testing of corneal sensitivity is very important for diagnosis of corneal diseases. No anesthetic agent is used while testing corneal sensitivity. It is done by two methods:

1. Make the patient sit on a stool comfortably. Ask him to keep looking straight with wide open eyes. Take sterile cotton and make it into a wick with very fine tip. Bring the cotton wick from behind the patient and touch the cornea at various points. Note down the blinking. Compare it with other eye using a different wick. Normally when cornea is touched with a cotton wick; patient blinks. However if corneal sensitivity is decreased; blinking is also decreased proportionately. This is the most common method employed clinically to test the sensitivity of cornea.
2. An *esthesiometer* is an instrument with a fine nylon tip **(Fig. 12.7)**. Instead of cotton wick this is used to test the corneal sensitivity. Different amount of pressure can be used to touch the cornea and notice blink reflex. Accordingly more is the pressure required to elicit blink reflex, lesser is the sensitivity of cornea.

CONJUNCTIVAL SWAB FOR CULTURE AND SENSITIVITY

It is taken in cases of infective conjunctivitis to identify the pathogen and the antibiotic, which would be effective against the infecting organism.

An autoclaved swab stick is taken and swept in the conjunctival fornix. It gets soaked in the conjunctival discharge. This discharge is applied over appropriate agar and incubated at desired temperature.

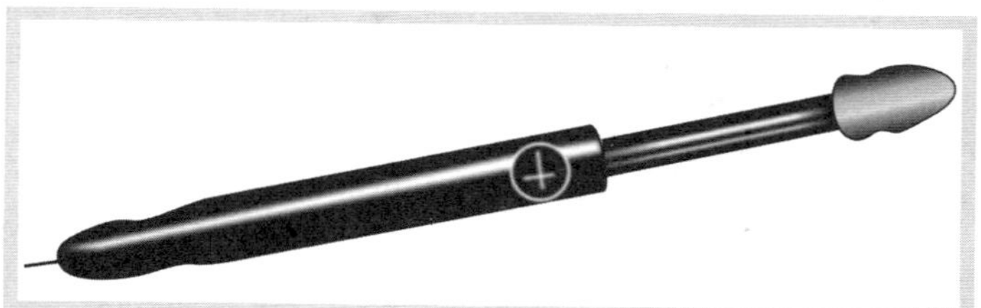

Fig. 12.7: Esthesiometer.

Any growth seen after 24–48 hours of incubation is tested to identify the pathogen. Sensitivity of antibiotics is also tested. This is done by making the bacteria grow on an appropriate agar along with an antibiotic. Commonly used antibiotics are applied on the agar at different places along with the bacterial growth. It is incubated at appropriate temperature for 24 hours. If a particular antibiotic is effective against bacteria, there will be no growth seen in the area of the antibiotic. Growth of bacteria in the vicinity of antibiotic shows that the particular antibiotic is not effective against that bacteria. Treatment of patient can be altered as per the reports of the test.

FUNDUS CAMERA

A fundus camera is a low power microscope type device used to take photographs of retina in different conditions **(Figs. 12.8A and B)**. It is used to diagnose a retinal disease and monitor its progression. It works on the principle of indirect ophthalmoscopy. It gives an upright, magnified view of the fundus. It views 30–50° of retinal area.

Clinical applications:

- Photograph of retina is taken to diagnose diseases like diabetic retinopathy, Eales' disease, primary open angle glaucoma, etc.
- Fundus fluorescein angiography is done to diagnose areas of non perfusion and any leakage of blood from retinal vessels.

Progress of a disease like glaucoma, diabetic retinopathy can be monitored by taking serial photographs at different periods of time.

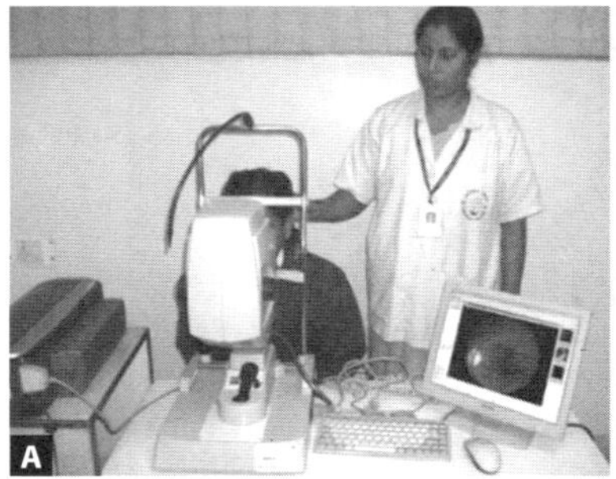

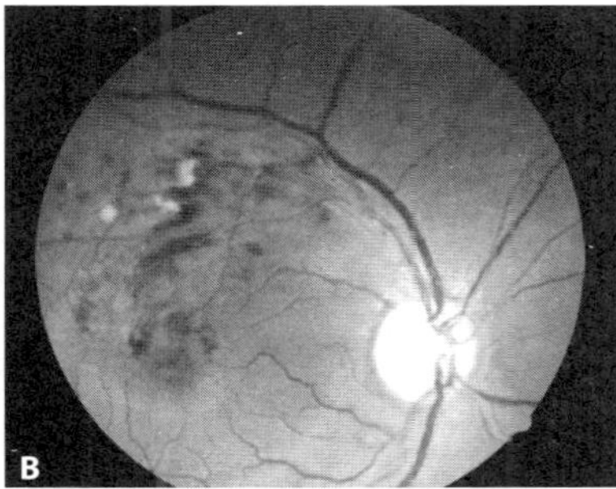

Figs. 12.8A and B: (A) Fundus camera; (B) Fundus photograph *(For color version, see Plate 2).*

FUNDUS FLUORESCEIN ANGIOGRAPHY

Fundus fluorescein angiography (FFA) is a procedure, which allows us to diagnose and manage various types of retinal disorders **(Fig. 12.9)**.

Indications of FFA

1. Diabetic retinopathy
2. Vaso-occlusive disorders
3. Eales' disease
4. Central serous retinopathy
5. Cystoid macular edema

Technique

Pupils of both eyes are dilated. Patient is seated against fundus camera. 3 mL 20% or 5 mL 10% sodium fluorescein dye is injected aseptically in antecubital vein and serial photography of fundus is done. First photograph is taken after 5 seconds, then every second for 20 seconds and then every 2–3 seconds for one minute. Photography is done for both eyes. Last picture is taken after 30 minutes.

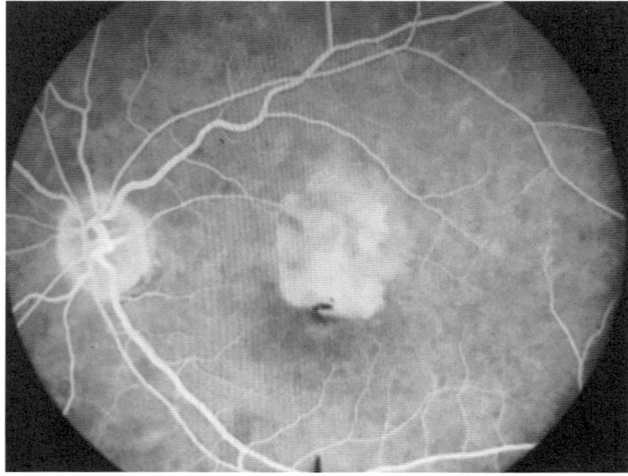

Fig. 12.9: Fundus angiogram.

Side Effects

It is a relatively safe procedure. However patient may develop allergic reaction to dye like nausea, vomiting, rashes and anaphylactic shock. A pre filled syringe of dexamethasone and chlorpheniramine maleate (CPM) should be ready to face such emergencies. All patients complain of yellowish discoloration of skin and urine.

This dye is nephrotoxic. So this procedure should not be done in nephro compromised patients as the dye is excreted in urine.

Phases of FFA

1. **Pre-arterial phase:** There is no dye in the circulation.
2. **Arterial phase:** Dye can be seen in arterioles.
3. **Arteriovenous phase:** Some dye can be seen in both arterioles and venules.
4. **Venous phase:** There is no dye in arterioles. It can be seen in venules.

Abnormalities Detected by FFA

FFA detects two types of abnormalities namely:

1. **Hypofluorescence:** Various causes are occlusion of blood vessels, hemorrhage or exudates.
2. **Hyperfluorescence:** Various causes are damage to RPE, pooling of dye as occurs in CME, CSR and microaneurysms.

FFA gives a very peculiar pattern in some diseases like inkblot appearance and smoke stack appearance in CSR and flower petal appearance in CME. Thus, FFA is very important tool for diagnosis and management of fundus disorders.

PLACIDO DISK

It is a disk painted with alternating black and white circles **(Fig. 12.10)**. It is used to check the regularity of corneal surface. Looking through the hole in the center of the disk a uniform sharp image of circles is seen on the cornea. If the corneal surface is irregular, circles appear distorted. However, with the advent of more sophisticated tests like corneal topography and pentacam this test is no more used clinically.

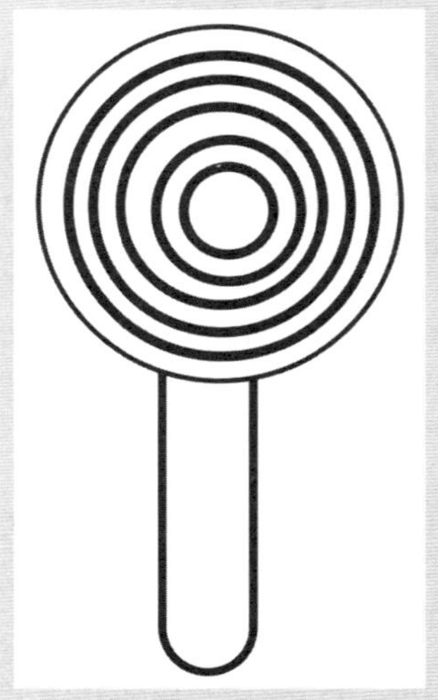

Fig. 12.10: Placido disk.

KERATOMETRY (OPHTHALMOMETRY)

It is a procedure by which we can measure the curvature of central part (2–4 mm) of anterior surface of cornea. The instrument is known as keratometer.

Uses

- It is used to calculate curvature of central part of cornea on its anterior surface. This curvature is used to calculate base curve of contact lens.
- It is also required to calculate power of IOL to be implanted after cataract surgery.
- Provides directions of principle meridia of cornea.
- Provides degree of corneal astigmatism.
- Provides information about any corneal surface distortion.

Principle

It is based on the principle that anterior surface of cornea acts as a convex mirror so the size of the image formed varies directly with curvature of cornea. Thus by knowing the size of image formed curvature of cornea can be calculated.

Types

Clinically, two types of keratometers are used:

1. **Javal Schiotz keratometer:** In this the target is like a step ladder. Horizontal and vertical curvatures cannot be measured simultaneously.
2. **Bausch and Lomb:** In this the target is in form of a circle and both horizontal and vertical curvatures can be measured simultaneously.

Depending upon operational technique, keratometers may be manual or autokeratometer **(Figs. 12.11 and 12.12)**.

Technique

- Look through eyepiece of keratometer and focus a black cross seen in the field.

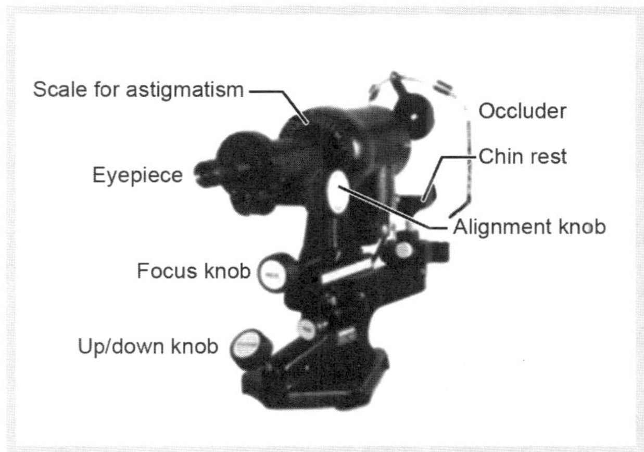

Fig. 12.11: Keratometer.

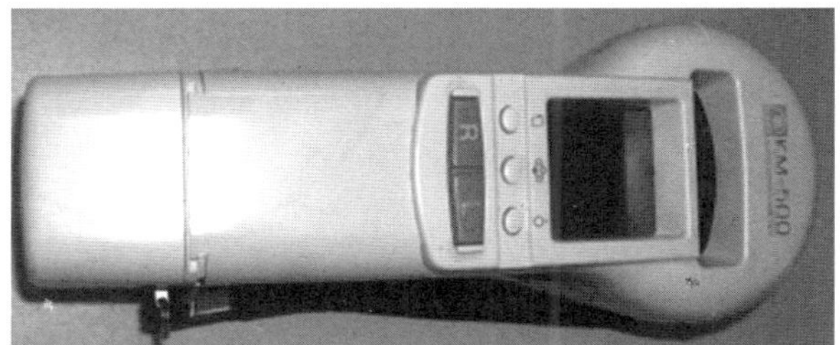

Fig. 12.12: Autokeratometer.

- Calibrate the instrument for any mechanical error.
- Make the patient sit on a stool comfortably and ask him to close the other eye. With the open eye he should see the illuminated target known as '*Mires*'. An image of circle is formed on his cornea (First Purkinje Image). If we look through eyepiece we see three mires; one in the center, one horizontal and one vertical. Focus the mires by 'focus knob' so that they look very sharp. Plus sign is seen in horizontal meridian near horizontal and central mires and minus sign is seen near vertical mire and central mire on vertical side. Adjust the horizontal and vertical knobs to align these minus and plus signs. Make sure the black cross is in the central mire **(Fig. 12.13)**. Take reading and adjust mechanical error if any. This gives curvature of cornea in diopter and millimeters. Reading in dioptre is used for IOL power calculation and reading in millimeters is used for CL fitting.

Range of Keratometer

Normal range of B and L keratometer is from 36 D to 52 D. However, the range can be increased or decreased by placing +1.25 D lens or -1.00 D lens in front of keratometer. Use +1.25 DS lens in front of the objective of the keratometer and add +9.00 to the scale reading OR place -1.00 DS lens in front of the objective and substract 6.00 from the scale reading. This maneuver

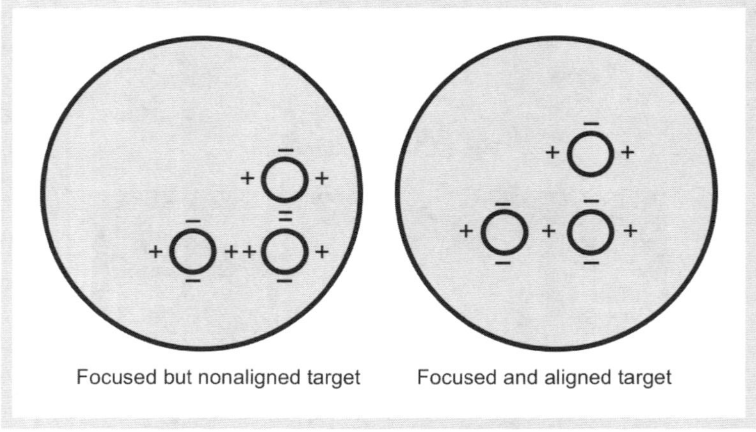

Fig. 12.13: Target of keratometer.

increases the range of the keratometer. Normal curvature of cornea is usually around +42 D.

Manual keratometer is preferred in patients with poor fixation, corneal abnormalities, distorted mires, high corneal astigmatism and dry eyes.

Sources of Error

- If we do not focus the black cross, it can introduce error of about 0.25 D.
- Noncalibration of instrument may be a source of big or small errors.
- Improper focusing and improper alignment of mires can be a source of error.

Note: Keratometry should always be performed prior to any procedure that requires local anesthesia like tonometry, pachymetry, biometry or any such applanation procedures because putting a local anesthetic agent over cornea causes corneal epithelial edema and keratometry becomes difficult as the mires become distorted.

BIOMETRY

It is a procedure by which we measure the power of intraocular lens to be implanted during cataract surgery to achieve desired post operative refractive status. It involves two procedures:

1. Keratometry
2. A-scan

First of all, Keratometry is done and findings are recorded. Axial length is measured with A-scan and the following formula is used:

$$\text{IOL power} = A - 2.5L - 0.9K;$$

where A = A constant of IOL
L = Axial length of eyeball
K = Keratometry reading

A-scan: Also called axial length scan. Axial length is measured in following cases:

1. IOL power calculation
2. High refractive error as a part of Myopia Control Programme.

It can be done with instruments like ultrasound A-scan, B-scan, optical biometer and IOL master.

Ultrasound A-scan: In cases of dense media opacities, ultrasound A-scan is useful. Ultrasound has an advantage over light as it has better penetration than the later.

For A-scan paracain eye drops are instilled in the eye of the patient to achieve topical anesthesia. Axial length of the eyeball is measured by touching the scan probe to the centre of cornea. Multiple readings are taken and the reading with good graph, i.e., where all the junctional spikes are of same height is selected. The standard deviation of readings should remain between 0.03–0.05. This reading along with findings of keratometry is fed into the formula and IOL power is calculated. This also requires 'A' constant value which is provided with the IOL by the company. The commonly used formulae are SRK II, SRK-T, Holladay, etc.

Techniques of A-scan Biometry

As on today A-scan biometry can be done by three techniques.

1. Contact biometry
2. Immersion biometry
3. Optical biometry

In **contact biometry** patient is seated comfortably on stool or made to lie down on bed.

Ultrasonic probe is made to touch the cornea after instillation of proparacaine eye drops. The axial length is displayed on the A-scan display screen. This technique has the disadvantage of touching the cornea and hence, some amount of pressure is exerted on the cornea which tends to under estimate axial length. Also there might be some injury to the cornea caused by the probe. Chances of infection are also there. However, this had been the most common technique of axial length measurement until immersion biometer and optical biometer replaced it.

A-scan biometer consists of a handheld probe which contains ultrasound transducer in it. It emits high-frequency ultrasonic waves that pass through cornea, AC, lens, vitreous and strike retina. From retina the waves are reflected back and received by the transducer. Time taken by the waves to travel ocular structures and back to the transducer is measured. As we know the speed of ultrasonic waves in different ocular media, hence, the distance between cornea and retina (axial length) can be calculated **(Figs. 12.14 and 12.15)**.

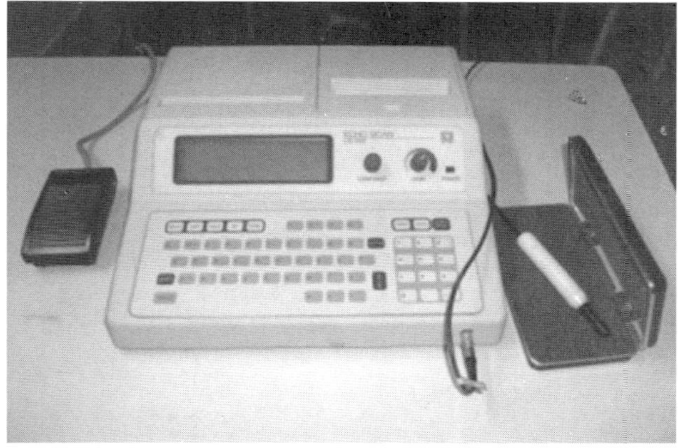

Fig. 12.14: A-scan.

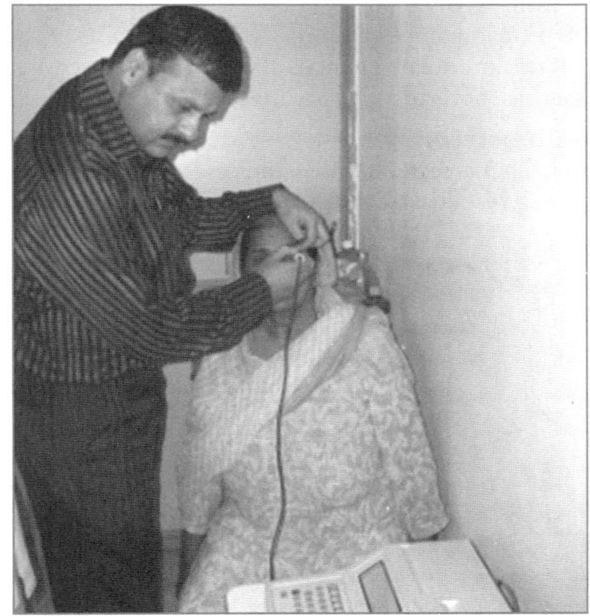

Fig. 12.15: Procedure of biometry.

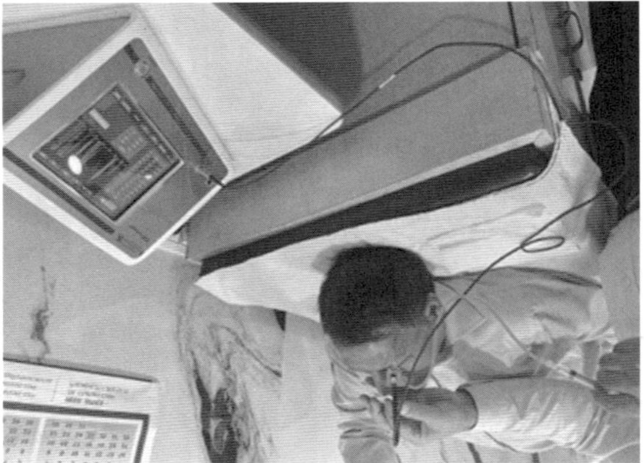

Fig. 12.16: Immersion biometry.

In **immersion biometry (Fig. 12.16)**, the ultrasonic probe is made to fit in a cup which is fitted on the cornea of the patient after making it numb with proparacaine eye drops. The cup contains normal saline solution. Here there are no chances of pressure on the cornea, hence, measurement is more accurate as compared to contact technique.

In **optical biometry**, patient is seated against the machine **(Fig. 12.17)**. Chin is rested on the chin rest and forehead is touched to the forehead rest. Just by clicking the specific knob, measurements

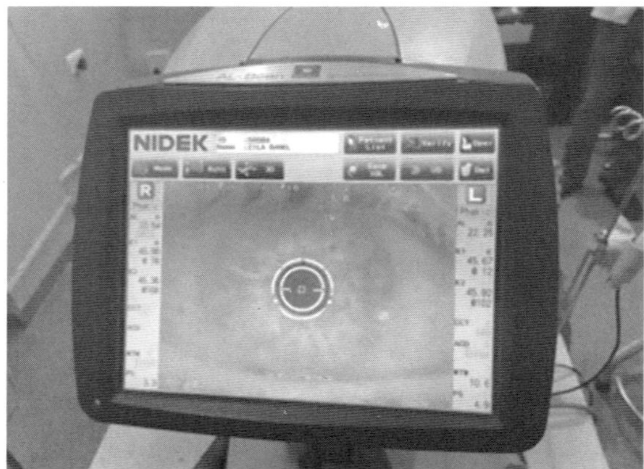

Fig. 12.17: Optical biometer.

are made and displayed on the screen. It is a very fast method, more accurate than contact biometry or immersion biometry and there are no chances of infection or underestimation as the cornea remains untouched. In addition, some other parameters of eyeball like anterior chamber depth, lens thickness, vitreous length, white to white diameter, corneal curvature, etc., are also measured by optical biometry.

Optical biometer works on the principle of partial coherence interferometry (PCI). It emits low coherence laser beam into the eye. The beam is split into two parts, one of which enters ocular structures and the other acts as a reference. After interacting with the eye, the two beams recombine and create interference patterns. These patterns are captured by the detector and analyzed using the software. By analyzing the patterns, the time taken by light waves to travel through ocular media and the speed of light in the ocular media, we can easily calculate the accurate axial length of the eyeball. With the introduction of premium IOLs, optical biometry is the only way to get accurate results, however it is very costly as compared to A-scan biometry or immersion biometry.

IOL master (Figs.12.18A and B): This is a very popular method of axial length measurement based on principles of optical biometry. In this method, optical coherent light passes through the visual axis and reflects back from the retinal pigment epithelium rather than

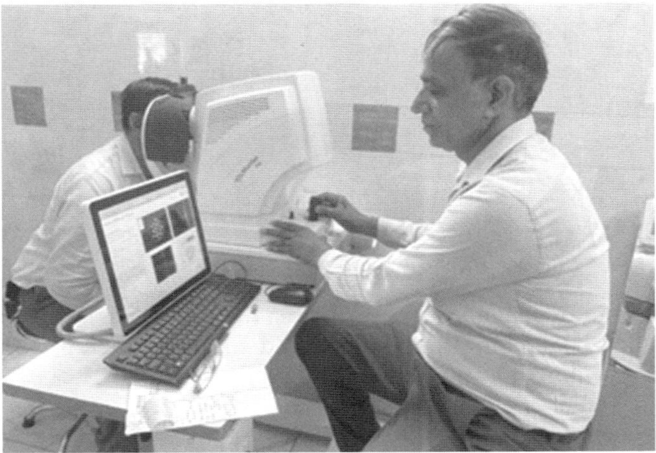

Fig. 12.18A: IOL master.

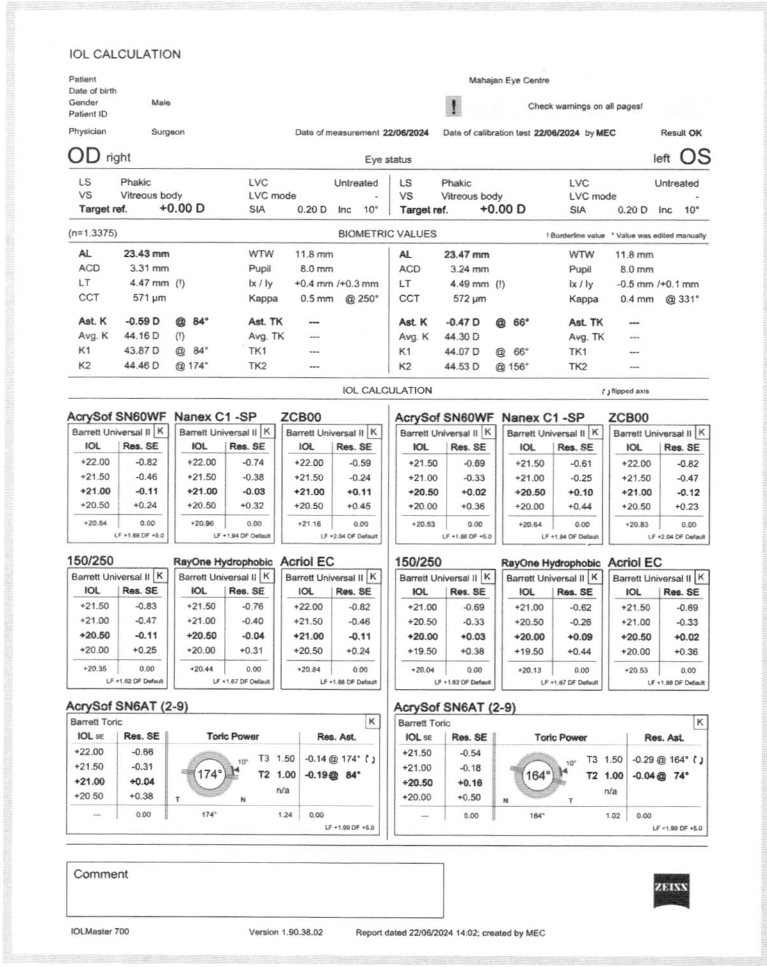

IOL CALCULATION

Patient
Date of birth
Gender Male
Patient ID

Mahajan Eye Centre

! Check warnings on all pages!

Physician Surgeon | Date of measurement 22/06/2024 | Date of calibration test 22/06/2024 by MEC | Result OK

OD right | Eye status | left OS

OD		LVC	Untreated	OS		LVC	Untreated
LS	Phakic	LVC mode	-	LS	Phakic	LVC mode	-
VS	Vitreous body	SIA	0.20 D Inc 10°	VS	Vitreous body	SIA	0.20 D Inc 10°
Target ref.	+0.00 D			Target ref.	+0.00 D		

(n=1.3375) BIOMETRIC VALUES ! Borderline value * Value was edited manually

OD				OS			
AL	23.43 mm	WTW	11.8 mm	AL	23.47 mm	WTW	11.8 mm
ACD	3.31 mm	Pupil	8.0 mm	ACD	3.24 mm	Pupil	8.0 mm
LT	4.47 mm (!)	Ix / Iy	+0.4 mm /+0.3 mm	LT	4.49 mm (!)	Ix / Iy	-0.5 mm /+0.1 mm
CCT	571 µm	Kappa	0.5 mm @ 250°	CCT	572 µm	Kappa	0.4 mm @ 331°
Ast. K	-0.59 D @ 84°	Ast. TK	---	Ast. K	-0.47 D @ 66°	Ast. TK	---
Avg. K	44.16 D (!)	Avg. TK	---	Avg. K	44.30 D	Avg. TK	---
K1	43.87 D @ 84°	TK1	---	K1	44.07 D @ 66°	TK1	---
K2	44.46 D @ 174°	TK2	---	K2	44.53 D @ 156°	TK2	---

IOL CALCULATION ( ) flipped axis

OD (right)

AcrySof SN60WF (Barrett Universal II) IOL	Res. SE	Nanex C1 -SP (Barrett Universal II) IOL	Res. SE	ZCB00 (Barrett Universal II) IOL	Res. SE
+22.00	-0.82	+22.00	-0.74	+22.00	-0.59
+21.50	-0.46	+21.50	-0.38	+21.50	-0.24
+21.00	-0.11	+21.00	-0.03	+21.00	+0.11
+20.50	+0.24	+20.50	+0.32	+20.50	+0.45
+20.84	0.00	+20.96	0.00	+21.16	0.00
	LF +1.88 DF +5.0		LF +1.94 DF Default		LF +2.04 DF Default

150/250 (Barrett Universal II) IOL	Res. SE	RayOne Hydrophobic (Barrett Universal II) IOL	Res. SE	Acriol EC (Barrett Universal II) IOL	Res. SE
+21.50	-0.83	+21.50	-0.76	+22.00	-0.82
+21.00	-0.47	+21.00	-0.40	+21.50	-0.46
+20.50	-0.11	+20.50	-0.04	+21.00	-0.11
+20.00	+0.25	+20.00	+0.31	+20.50	+0.24
+20.35	0.00	+20.44	0.00	+20.84	0.00
	LF +1.62 DF Default		LF +1.67 DF Default		LF +1.88 DF Default

AcrySof SN6AT (2-9) — Barrett Toric

IOL SE	Res. SE	Toric Power		Res. Ast.
+22.00	-0.66	T3	1.50	-0.14 @ 174° ( )
+21.50	-0.31	T2	1.00	-0.19 @ 84°
+21.00	+0.04		n/a	
+20.50	+0.38			
---	0.00	174°	1.24	0.00
				LF +1.99 DF +5.0

OS (left)

AcrySof SN60WF (Barrett Universal II) IOL	Res. SE	Nanex C1 -SP (Barrett Universal II) IOL	Res. SE	ZCB00 (Barrett Universal II) IOL	Res. SE
+21.50	-0.69	+21.50	-0.61	+22.00	-0.82
+21.00	-0.33	+21.00	-0.25	+21.50	-0.47
+20.50	+0.02	+20.50	+0.10	+21.00	-0.12
+20.00	+0.36	+20.00	+0.44	+20.50	+0.23
+20.53	0.00	+20.64	0.00	+20.83	0.00
	LF +1.88 DF +5.0		LF +1.94 DF Default		LF +2.04 DF Default

150/250 (Barrett Universal II) IOL	Res. SE	RayOne Hydrophobic (Barrett Universal II) IOL	Res. SE	Acriol EC (Barrett Universal II) IOL	Res. SE
+21.00	-0.69	+21.00	-0.62	+21.50	-0.69
+20.50	-0.33	+20.50	-0.26	+21.00	-0.33
+20.00	+0.03	+20.00	+0.09	+20.50	+0.02
+19.50	+0.38	+19.50	+0.44	+20.00	+0.36
+20.04	0.00	+20.13	0.00	+20.53	0.00
	LF +1.62 DF Default		LF +1.67 DF Default		LF +1.88 DF Default

AcrySof SN6AT (2-9) — Barrett Toric

IOL SE	Res. SE	Toric Power		Res. Ast.
+21.50	-0.54	T3	1.50	-0.29 @ 164° ( )
+21.00	-0.18	T2	1.00	-0.04 @ 74°
+20.50	+0.16		n/a	
+20.00	+0.50			
---	0.00	164°	1.02	0.00
				LF +1.99 DF +5.0

Comment

ZEISS

IOLMaster 700 | Version 1.90.38.02 | Report dated 22/06/2024 14:02; created by MEC

Fig. 12.18B: Printout of IOL master.

internal limiting membrane like in other methods. This factor should be compensated and the result should coincide to an immersion A-scan to within 0.1 mm.

Advantages

- It is known for its accurate and quick measurements, hence, enhancing surgeon and patient experience.

- It is a noncontact technique. Hence, there are no chances of infection or injury to cornea.
- It is compatible with latest IOLs like toric, multifocal IOLs, incorporating all types of formula required for IOL calculation like eye with silicone oil, pseudophakic eyes, aphakic eyes, post -LASIK and post-RK eyes, etc.
- It gives the refractive axial length versus the anatomic axial length achieved with ultrasound biometry.
- It also measures corneal curvatures, anterior chamber depth, White to white diameter (limbus to limbus diameter used in ICL implantation), central corneal thickness, angle kappa, pupil size and lens thickness in addition to the axial length.

Disadvantages

- Inability to measure through dense cataracts and other media opacities, like corneal opacity because light cannot penetrate opaque medium.
- Accuracy is compromised in patients with nystagmus, tremors when patient is not able to fixate properly.
- Important sources of error are corneal scars or dystrophies that create an irregular anterior corneal surface.

B-scan: It uses high-frequency sound waves (ultrasound) to create cross sectional images of lens, vitreous, retina, etc. Hence, vitreous hemorrhage, retinal detachment, intraocular tumors can be easily visualized.

CORNEAL TOPOGRAPHY

Also known as photokeratoscopy or videokeratography is a noninvasive technique for mapping the curvature of anterior surface of cornea. This is a three-dimensional map valuable in the:

- Diagnosis of early keratoconus
- Assessing fitting of semisoft contact lens
- In planning LASIK laser surgery
- Evaluation of irregular
- Astigmatism especially after penetrating keratoplasty
- Planning of removal of sutures after surgery

It is an OPD procedure, carried out in seconds and is completely painless.

Principle

Multiple light concentric rings are projected on the cornea. The reflected image is captured on a charge-coupled device camera. Computer software analyzes the data and displays the results in different formats.

Normal cornea flattens from center toward periphery by 2D–4D, nasal area flattening more than the temporal area. Corneal topography of two corneas of an individual often shows mirror image symmetry. Common patterns seen in topography are round, oval, symmetric bow tie for regular astigmatism, asymmetric bow tie and irregular. The topography is depicted with warm and cool colors. The flatter cornea is depicted by green and steeper corneas show shades of yellow and orange.

PENTACAM (FIGS. 12.19A AND B)

It is another very important latest technological advancement in the mapping of both anterior and posterior surfaces of cornea. It is superior to corneal topography as it gives high resolution images of the entire cornea including calculation of pachymetry from limbus to limbus. Corneal topography tells us about the abnormalities of anterior surface of cornea only but pentacam can detect

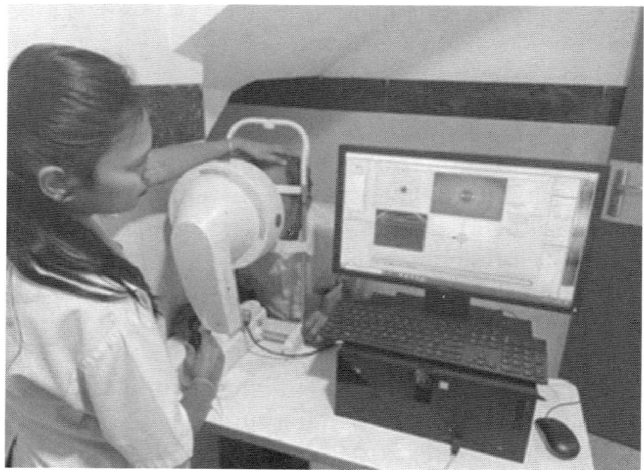

Fig. 12.19A: A pentacam machine.

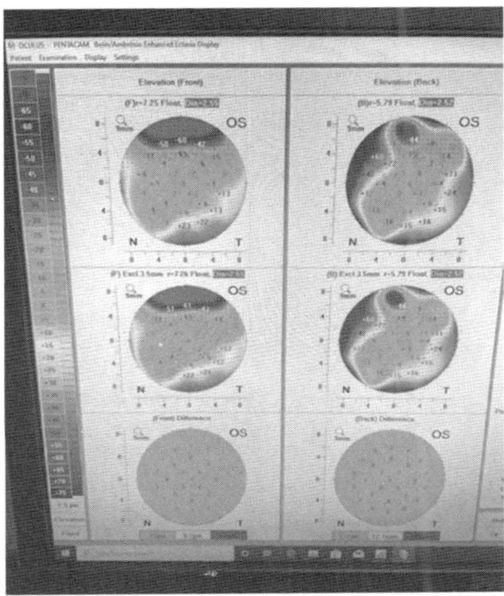

Fig. 12.19B: Pentacam image.

abnormalities of both anterior and posterior surface of cornea. It can also provide corneal wavefront analysis to detect higher order aberrations.

Orbscan is another latest instrument used in clinical practice to analyze the thickness and the entire posterior surface of cornea.

GENEVA LENS MEASURE (FIG.12.20)

It is a pocket watch-shaped instrument used to measure the power of a curved surface like a convex or concave lens. Power can be measured in different meridians. There are three-pointed prongs attached to the instrument one of them (middle one) is movable and other two being fixed. When we place the watch on a curved surface, the movable prong is displaced by the curvature of the curved surface which is reflected in the calibrated scale on the watch. The algebraic sum of readings of both the surfaces gives the net power of the lens. Thus, power of both spherical and cylindrical lens along with its axis can be measured by the instrument. This instrument is calibrated for lenses made of crown glass with refractive index of 1.523 and reading is recorded in Diopters. Power of lenses made of other material with different refractive index can also be calculated from a formula **(Fig. 12.20)**.

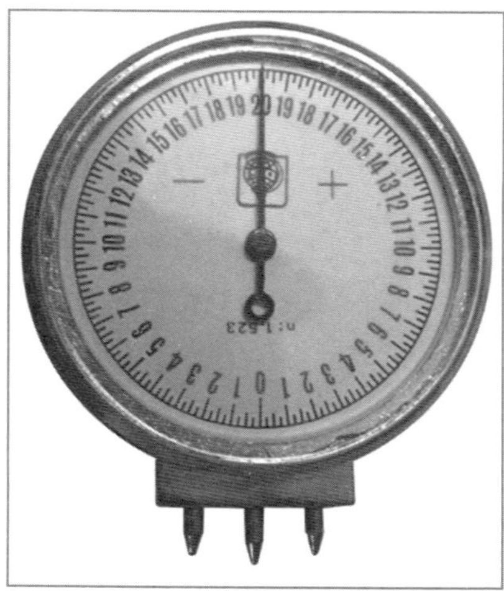

Fig. 12.20: Geneva lens measure.

OPTICAL COHERENCE TOMOGRAPHY (FIGS. 12.21A TO C)

It is a noninvasive method clinically used for imaging of retina. Similar to CT scan of internal organs, OCT uses the optical backscattering of light to rapidly scan the eye and describe a pixel representation of the anatomic layers of retina. It is an interferometric

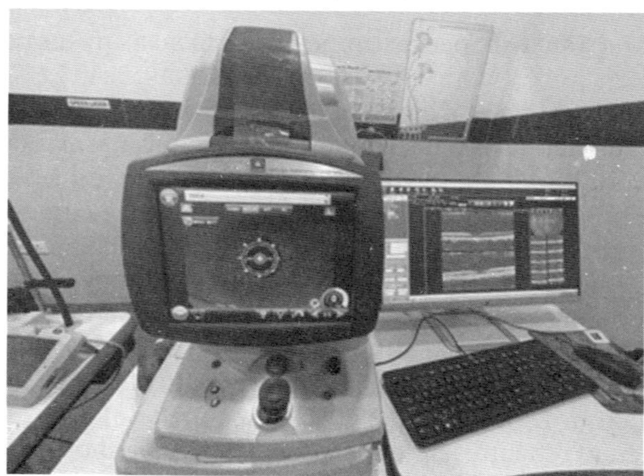

Fig. 12.21A: OCT machine.

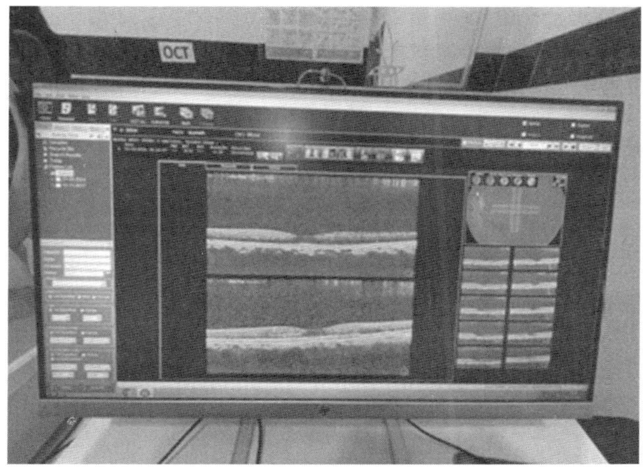

Fig. 12.21B: OCT image.

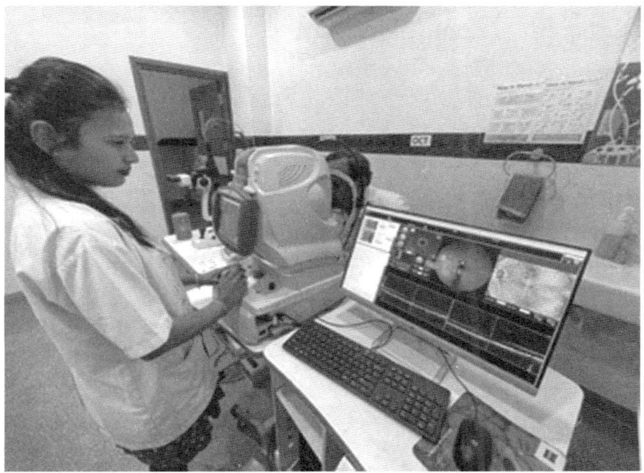

Fig. 12.21C: OCT procedure.

technique using near infrared light. The greater wavelength of light used makes it able to penetrate better into the scattering medium. All the ten layers of retina can be differentiated and their thickness can be measured. Confocal microscopy is another similar technique but with less penetration.

Clinically, certain conditions like age related macular degeneration and cystoid macular edema can be diagnosed eliminating the need for FFA. This technique has achieved sub-micrometer resolutions.

SYNOPTOPHORE (FIG. 12.22)

This is an instrument used for:

- Detection and measurement of latent squint (heterophoria)
- Detection and measurement of manifest squint (heterotropia)
- Convergence and divergence exercises
- Measurement of subjective and objective angles of deviation
- To detect retinal correspondence, harmonious and unharmonious.
- Detection of grades of binocular single vision.
- Orthoptic exercises to develop BSV in patients who do not have BSV.
- To detect presence and type of suppression.
- Measurement of IPD.
- Measurement of angle alpha.
- Measurement of range of fusion.

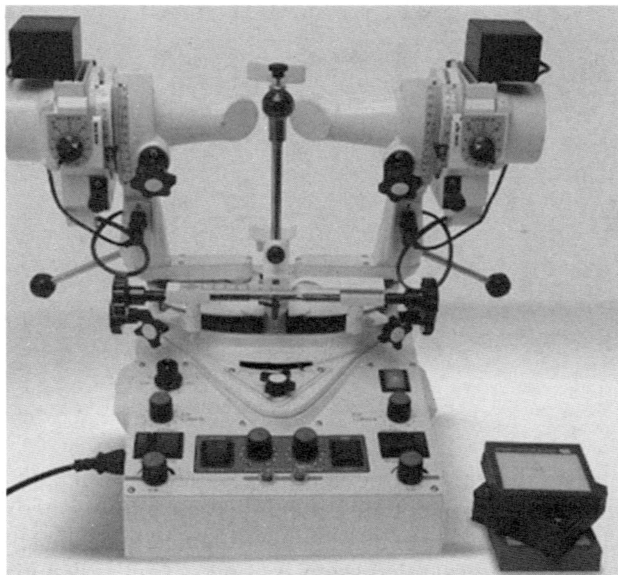

Fig. 12.22: Synoptophore.

It has one disadvantage that measurement for distance is not accurate because even when the instrument is set for distance psychic convergence comes into play and vitiates the measurements.

The instrument consists of base unit with illuminating system, slide holders, reflecting mirrors and lenses. Separate screws are provided for adjusting vertical and torsional deviations. Each eyepiece contains +6.50 DS lens to relax the accommodation completely. Interpupillary distance is adjustable. Tubes can be moved from a convergence position of 50° to a divergence position of 40°. The illuminating system is so constructed that there is no intense reflection. The intensity of light can be adjusted by rheostats. Slides are inserted at the ends of the tubes. There is also a slot for using Haidinger brushes in the two arms of the synoptophore. Arrangement for putting the light off in front of any of the slide carriers is available. This system can be utilized for rapid flashing of light for stimulating the under functioning macula.

OPHTHALMOSCOPY

It is a method by which we see the details of the fundus and detect opacities in the media. It is of three types:

1. Distant direct ophthalmoscopy
2. Direct ophthalmoscopy
3. Indirect ophthalmoscopy

Distant Direct Ophthalmoscopy

This procedure should be routinely performed before direct ophthalmoscopy. This is the best method to detect opacities in the media. It can be performed by a direct ophthalmoscope or a plane mirror with a hole in the center (plane retinoscope) or even a concave retinoscope or indirect ophthalmoscope **(Fig. 12.23)**.

Technique

Throw light on eyeball of patient from a distance of 20–25 cm in a dark room and observe the pupil. Pupil appears red in color under normal circumstances.

Clinical Applications

- **To detect opacities in the media:** Any opacity in the media appears as a black shadow against red fundal glow. Ask the patient

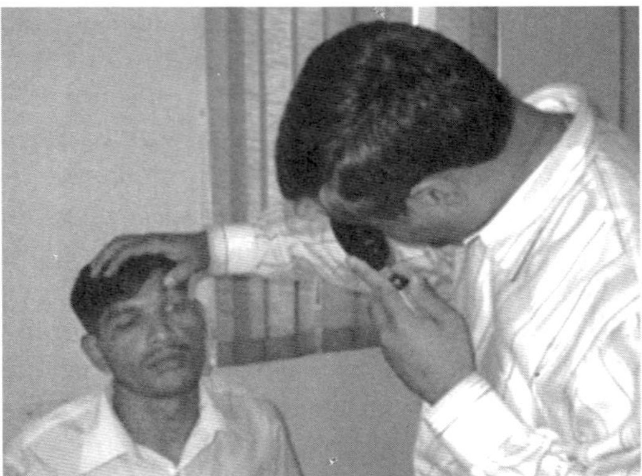

Fig. 12.23: Distant direct ophthalmoscopy.

to move his eye right-left and up-down. Observe the movement of opacity. Opacities in the pupillary plane show no movement, opacities in front of pupillary plane (e.g., in AC) move with the movement of eyeball and those behind the pupillary plane (e.g., in the vitreous) move against the movement of eyeball.

- **To differentiate between a hole and a mole:** A hole in the iris is like a peripheral iridectomy and a mole on the iris both appear black in color. On DDO, a red glow is seen through the hole but a mole remains black in color.
- **To suspect a detached retina/tumor of fundus:** A grayish reflex is seen in the pupil if the retina is detached or there is a tumor arising from the fundus.

Direct Ophthalmoscopy

It is done with direct ophthalmoscope **(Figs. 12.24 and 12.25)**. This instrument is a handy, self illuminated instrument to view fundus details. It has two parts, a handle which contains rechargeable battery or disposable battery and the optical part called the head. Ophthalmoscope was invented by von Helmholtz in 1850.

Technique

Pupil of patient is dilated. Hold the ophthalmoscope in your right hand and examine the right eye of the patient with your right eye standing on the right side of the patient. See the red fundal glow.

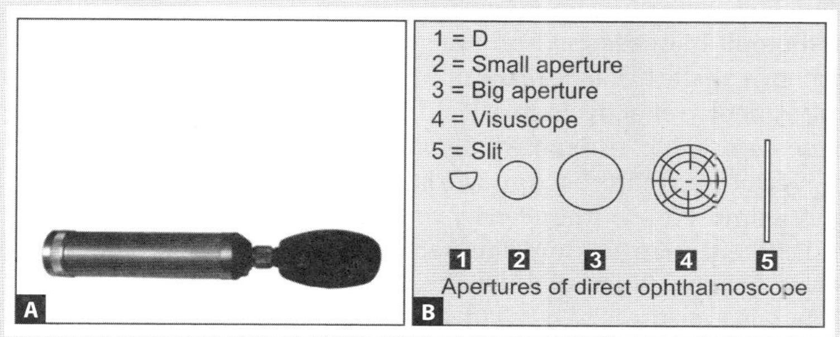

Figs. 12.24A and B: (A) Direct; (B) Indirect ophthalmoscope.

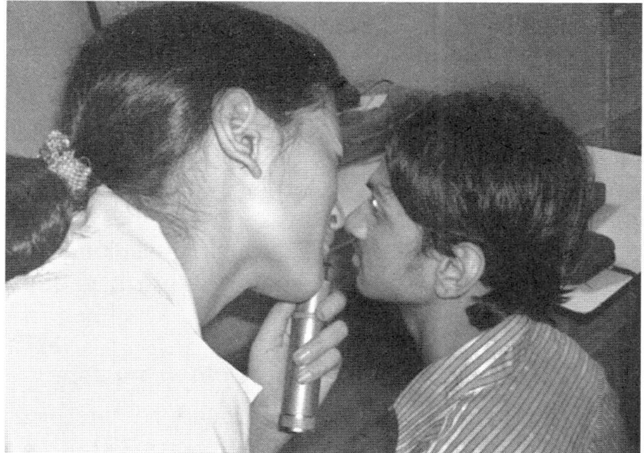

Fig. 12.25: Direct ophthalmoscopy.

Now go as close to the patient's eye as possible and focus any part of retina by moving lens wheel with index finger of your right hand. Trace any of the blood vessels toward its starting point and you will be able to reach the optic disk. If you ask the patient to look straight ahead, optic disk comes into focus. If patient sees the light of the instrument, macula comes into focus. Other details of fundus like blood vessels and background are also noted. Similarly, left eye of patient is examined with your left eye holding the instrument in your left hand and standing on the left side of the patient. Dioptric power of lens wheel required to examine the retina of patient depends on clinician's refractive status, patient's refractive status and the distance of the ophthalmoscope from the patient's cornea. The field of view depends on the distance of the ophthalmoscope from patient's cornea and patient's refractive status. Field of view is more as we approach the patient's eye. It is also more in hypermetropes than myopes.

Direct ophthalmoscope works on the principle of glass plate ophthalmoscope introduced by von Helmholtz.

Different apertures and filters are provided in the ophthalmoscope for performing different functions:

- Small aperture is to be used to examine the fundus through small undilated pupil. Similarly, medium and large apertures are used depending upon the size of the pupil.
- Visuscope or star or Graticule is used to see type of fixation. Patient is asked to focus on the light. If he is able to follow the star, it implies foveal fixation.
- Slit aperture is used to assess levels of lesions and tumors. It is also used to differentiate macular hole and macular cyst.
- Cobalt blue filter is used to see lesions of cornea after fluorescein staining.
- Red free filter (green filter) is used to see nerve fiber bundle defects in glaucoma, improve contrast in viewing retinal blood vessels and hemorrhages and to distinguish retinal hemorrhage from micro aneurysm.

Advantages and Disadvantages of Direct Ophthalmoscopy

It is easier to perform and master the procedure. Interpretation is also very easy as the image formed is erect. Image is 15× magnified, so minor details can be seen easily. However, it gives a monocular view and lacks depth perception. Because of high magnification, field of view is restricted. Examination of retina beyond equator is not possible.

Indirect Ophthalmoscopy

It is done with indirect ophthalmoscope **(Figs. 12.26A and B)**. This instrument is used to examine peripheral details of retina. Advantages of indirect ophthalmoscopy over direct ophthalmoscopy are **(Table 12.1)**:

- It gives binocular view hence is much better to detect shallow retinal detachments.

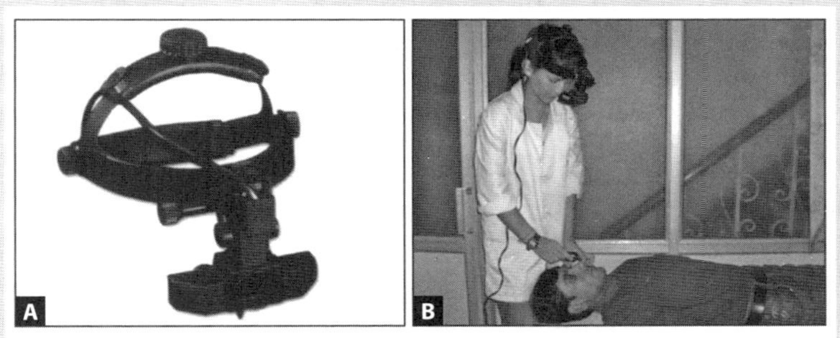

Figs. 12.26A and B: Indirect ophthalmoscopy.

Table 12.1: Comparison between direct and indirect ophthalmoscopes.

	Direct	*Indirect*
Image characteristics	Virtual, erect, 15× magnified but field of view is small (about 2 disk diameters) hence, comparison of two eyes is difficult	Real, inverted, magnified image, field of view much larger (about 8 disk diameters) hence, comparison is easy
Stereopsis	Not present	Present
Extent of retina examined	Up to equator	Up to ora serrata
Interpretation	Easy as the image is erect	Difficult because image formed is inverted and laterally reversed
Technique	Easy to master	Difficult to master
Examination through hazy media	Not possible as the illumination is lesser	Possible as the illumination is much brighter
Examination distance	As close to the eye of patient as possible	At an arm's length
Condensing lens	Not required	It is a must

- Field of view is bigger but magnification is less. Magnification depends upon power of lens used. With +20 D lens 3× magnification is achieved.
- It is easier to compare the retinal details of two eyes.
- Whole of the retina can be examined; up to ora serrata which is not possible with direct ophthalmoscope.

The *principle* of indirect ophthalmoscope is that eyeball is made highly myopic by interposing a high plus lens between the ophthalmoscope and the eyeball hence a real, inverted and laterally reversed, magnified image of retina is formed in the air between the lens and the eyeball.

Technique of Indirect Ophthalmoscopy

Make the patient lie down comfortably on examination table with pupil fully dilated. Hold the condensing lens in one hand and open the eye with other hand. Throw the light of ophthalmoscope on eyeball from an arm's length. Interpose the condensing lens close to the eye of the patient. Move the lens away from eyeball slowly till the retina comes into view. Now focus the view and examine it. Ask the patient to move his eyes right, left, up and down to examine the periphery. Scleral depression is required to examine the extreme periphery of the retina. Findings can be noted by drawing fundus diagram on paper using color codes.

GONIOSCOPY

It is a procedure by which we can see details of angle of anterior chamber **(Figs. 12.27A and B)**. It is an OPD procedure. It is done with an instrument called gonioscope. Different structures seen with a gonioscope are:

- **Schwalbe's line:** It is the termination of descemet's membrane. It appears as a solid, glistening structure.
- **Trabecular meshwork:** It gives soft, velvety appearance. It is easy to identify at 12 o'clock position due to its pigmentation. It has

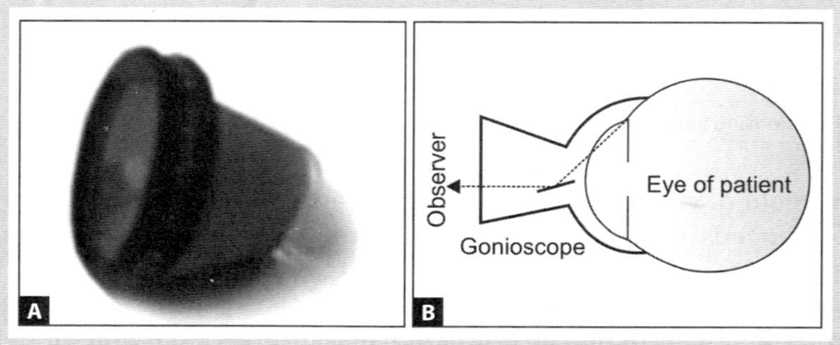

Figs. 12.27A and B: Gonioscope and its optics.

two parts: Anterior one-third is non-pigmented and posterior two-third parts is pigmented. Schlemm's canal is visible only if it is filled with blood.

- **Scleral spur:** It is a narrow, solid, whitish band, easily identified at 12 o'clock position where it is least likely to be covered with pigments. It is half the width of TM.
- **Ciliary body band:** It is as wide as the TM. In angle recession width of ciliary body band is more than width of TM.
- Iris processes can also be seen in young people. They need to be differentiated from peripheral anterior synechiae (PAS) when present. PAS are seen in angle closure glaucoma and are best seen in superior angles. PAS of inflammatory origin are best seen in inferior angles.

Clinical Application of Gonioscopy

- It is done to assess depth of angle of anterior chamber. Depth of angle of AC can be divided into four grades:
  - **Grade 0:** Iris is in contact with the corneal endothelium. No structure of angle can be seen. It is seen in acute angle closure attack. Immediate treatment is required to save vision.
  - **Grade 1:** Only Schwalbe's line is visible. There are high chances of angle getting closed hence immediate preventive measures need to be taken like YAG iridotomy.
  - **Grade 2:** Schwalbe's line and TM is visible. There are less chances of angle getting closed.
  - **Grade 3:** Schwalbe's line with TM and scleral spur are visible. It is an open angle and there are no chances of angle closure.
  - **Grade 4:** Schwalbe's line, TM, Scleral spur and ciliary body band are visible. It is a wide open angle and there are no chances of angle closure.
- Angle recession can be diagnosed only by doing gonioscopy.
- Gonioscopy is a must for diagnosis and treatment of congenital glaucoma.

Gonioscopy is of two types; namely direct and indirect gonioscopy. In direct gonioscopy structures are seen directly but in indirect gonioscopy mirror images of structures are seen, i.e., inferior angle is seen superiorly and right sided angle is seen on left side and vice versa. Koeppe, Barkan, Swan-Jacob and Thorpe goniolenses are examples of direct gonioscope and Goldmann three mirror gonioscopes, Zeiss 4-mirror goniolens are examples of indirect goniolens. Direct goniolens is more suitable for surgical procedures like goniotomy. Indirect goniolens is more com-monly used for classification of glaucoma.

Technique

Make the patient sit against slit lamp. Explain him the procedure properly. Put one drop of 2% xylocaine eye drop. Take the goniolens, put some coupling fluid like 2% HPMC and insert it over cornea. Using slit-lamp beam different angle structures can be seen. Examination of 360° angle can be done by rotating the goniolens 360° gradually. While using Goldmann three-mirror gonioscope dome-shaped mirror is used for gonioscopy. Structures can be seen more easily if during the procedure patient is asked to look toward the mirror of the goniolens.

PACHYMETER

It is an instrument used to measure the thickness of cornea. It is required prior to LASIK laser surgery, screening of keratoconus and monitoring of glaucoma. There are two types of pachymeters: Optical pachymeter and ultrasonic pachymeter. Ultrasonic pachymeters are the latest ones used clinically. It works by way of corneal waveform. It is just like A-scan of eyeball. It is accurate and can detect structures within corneal substance like microbubbles created in the cornea during femtosecond laser flap.

Procedure

Patient is seated on a stool. One drop of local anesthetic agent is put in the eye. Wait for 30 second for proper anesthesia. Take the probe and touch the central part of cornea perpendicularly and gently. Corneal thickness is displayed on monitor in micrometers. Multiple readings are taken and average is considered with SD within 0.03–0.05.

AMSLER GRID

This is a chart devised by Marc Amsler to detect slight abnormalities of central 20° of visual field. Most commonly used chart consists of

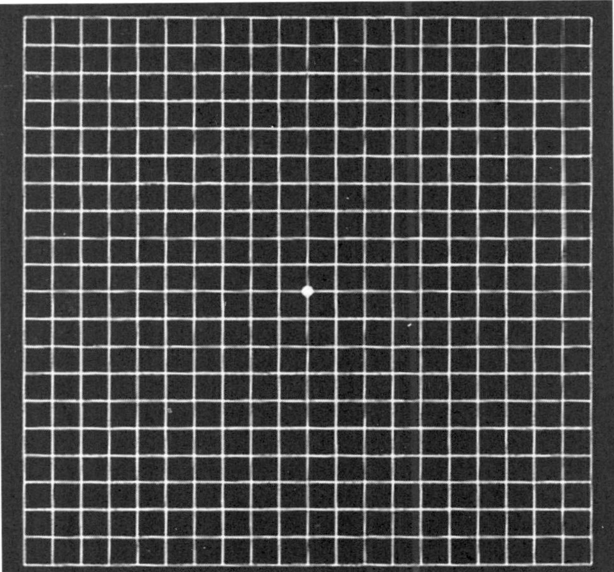

Fig. 12.28: Amsler grid.

a white grid of 5 mm squares on a black background with a central white fixation point **(Fig. 12.28)**.

Technique

Patient is seated comfortably in a well lit room. Patient should see this chart with best corrected vision, i.e., after using spectacles if required. Chart is held at a distance of 25 cm. No medicine should be used prior to this procedure so that accommodation is intact and there is no change in pupillary size. Patient is instructed to look at the fixation point of chart with one eye, other eye being closed. Ask the following questions:

1. Are you able to see the fixation point? If not it is due to presence of central scotoma.
2. With eyes seeing at fixation point can you see whole of the chart or any portion of chart is missing? It may be due to paracentral scotoma.
3. Is there any waviness in the horizontal or vertical lines? This may indicate metamorphopsia. It occurs if distance between two cones is altered as in macular edema.

4. Is there any blurred or distorted area in the grid? These changes appear prior to appearance of a definite scotoma.

VISUAL FIELD CHARTING (PERIMETRY)

This is a procedure by which we estimate extent of visual field. Visual field is a three-dimensional area around an object of regard (fixation point). Extent of visual field is 90° temporal, 60° nasal, 70° inferior and 60° superior with a white object of 5 mm size. Perimetry is of two types:

1. **Kinetic perimetry:** Here the stimulus is moved from periphery to center like confrontation method, tangent screen, etc.
2. **Static perimetry:** Here stimulus of known luminance is presented at preset positions for a preset duration. Automated perimetry is an example of static perimetry.

Central field can be charted with scotometry, Goldmann perimetry and automated field analyzer. Peripheral field can be charted with confrontation method, Lister's perimeter, Goldmann perimeter and automated perimeters.

Confrontation Method

Here visual field of examiner is compared with visual field of patient presuming that the visual field of examiner is normal. It is a very easy method and can be done anytime, anywhere without any instrumentation. Patient sits in front of the examiner at a distance of one meter. Patient closes his right eye and examiner closes his left eye. Thus visual field of left eye of patient is compared with visual field of right eye of examiner. Patient is asked to look into the right eye of examiner with his left eye. The examiner brings his finger from periphery to center midway between patient and himself. Both patient and examiner must see the finger simultaneously to consider the visual field of patient as normal.

Lister's Perimeter

It is used to estimate the extent of peripheral field. It consists of a metallic semicircular arc with a scale and a white dot for fixation. The arc can be rotated in different directions. Patient is asked to sit in front of the perimeter such that the chin is rested on the chin rest. One eye of patient is occluded at one time. He sees the fixation point with open eye. An object is moved from periphery to center till he

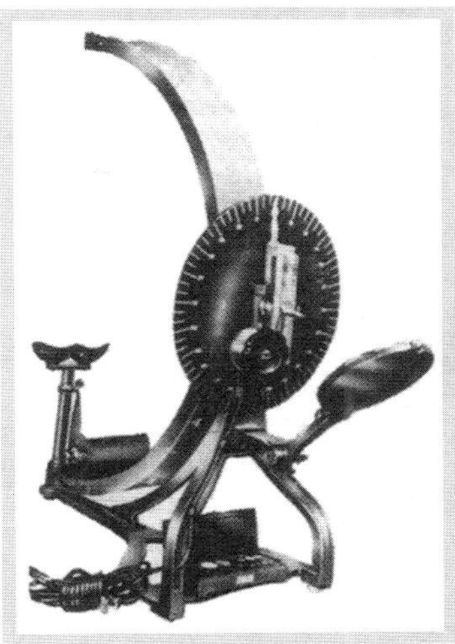

Fig. 12.29: Lister's perimeter.

starts appreciating the object. This point is noted on the scale. Similar recordings are done in different directions. Size and color of object is noted **(Fig. 12.29)**.

Scotometry

It is used to estimate central 30° field. The Bjerrum's screen is practically used for this purpose. It may be of one meter or two meter square size. Patient is seated at a distance of one and two meters respectively. Screen consists of a central fixation point around which are concentric circles from 5–30°. Patient is asked to fixate at the central dot with one eye, other eye being occluded. First of all, blind spot is charted with one eye. Then a white target of 10 mm size is moved from periphery to center in different directions and any point where the target becomes invisible is recorded. Blind spot is located about 15° temporal in the horizontal meridian. Central and paracentral scotomas can be found by this method **(Fig. 12.30)**.

Automated Perimeter

This is the current gold standard. Patient is seated against a concave dome with presbyopic correction if required. One eye of patient is occluded. Patient sees the central target with the open eye. Computer

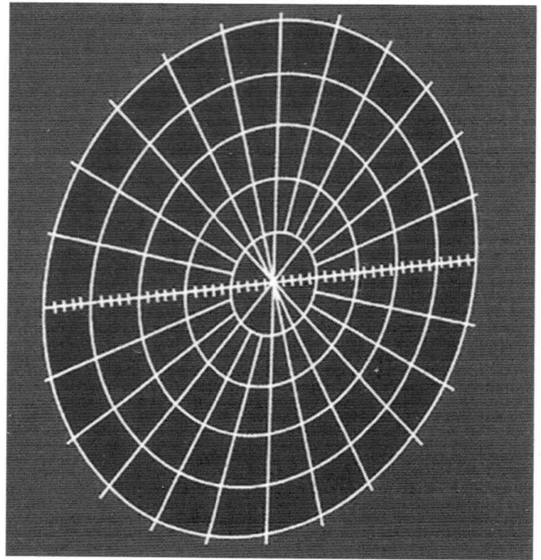

Fig. 12.30: Bjerrum's screen.

shines light at predetermined positions and of particular intensity. Patient is instructed to press a button whenever he sees a light at any point without loosing his fixation. Computer records this and compares it with the normal value for the age already fed in its software **(Figs. 12.31 and 12.32)**.

Scotoma

It is an area of partial alteration in the field of vision which consists of a partially diminished or entirely damaged visual acuity surrounded by a field of relatively normal vision. In simple words it is a partly or totally blind area in the visual field. It is of different types:

- **Physiological scotoma:** It is present in each and every individual, e.g., blind spot.
- **Pathological scotoma:** It indicates some abnormality of retina or optic nerve, e.g., arcuate scotoma, paracentral scotoma, central scotoma, etc.
- **Negative scotoma:** This type of scotoma cannot be appreciated by the patient himself but can be charted on perimetry. Blind spot is a negative scotoma. Thus this type of scotoma is a sign and not a symptom.

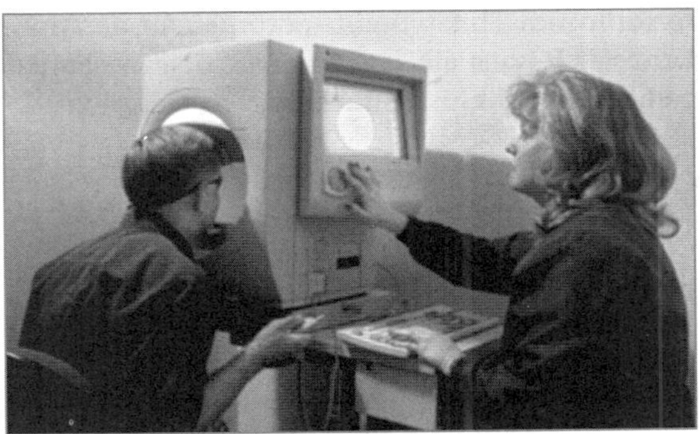

Fig.12.31: Automated perimeter.

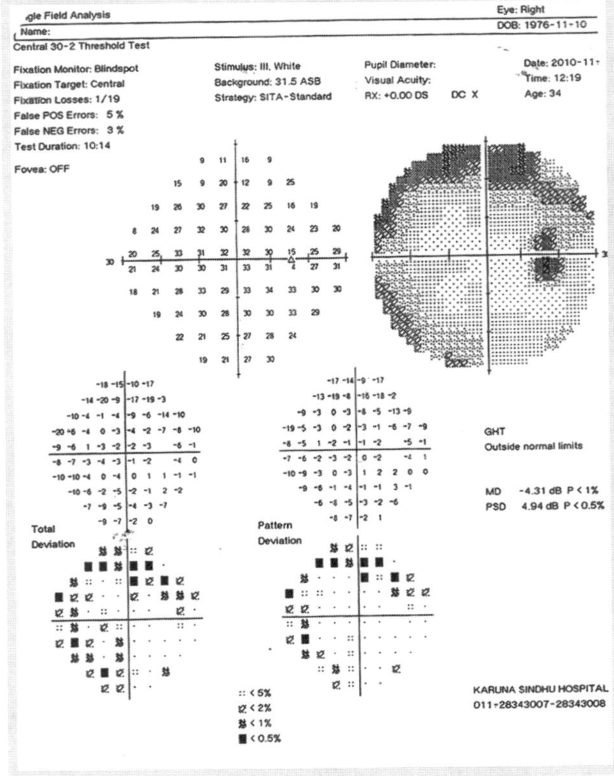

Fig. 12.32: Visual field chart.

- **Positive scotoma:** This type of scotoma can be appreciated by patient himself. It is usually late stage of a disease. Patient says that he sees a black spot in his visual field.

CONTRAST SENSITIVITY

Contrast is the difference in visual properties that makes an object distinguishable from other objects and the background. Contrast sensitivity is the ability of the eye to see objects that may not be outlined clearly or that do not stand out from their background, e.g., ability to appreciate a gray object against a white background. Contrast sensitivity is maximum at 20 years of age and at spatial frequencies of about 2–5 cycles/degree. It decreases with age, in cataract, and diabetic retinopathy **(Fig. 12.33)**.

Clinical Features of Low Contrast Sensitivity

- Difficulty in seeing traffic lights or vehicles at night.
- Not able to see a burning flame on stove.
- A very good illumination is required to read or write.
- Not able to see spots on cloths or dishes.
- Feeling of tiredness while watching TV.

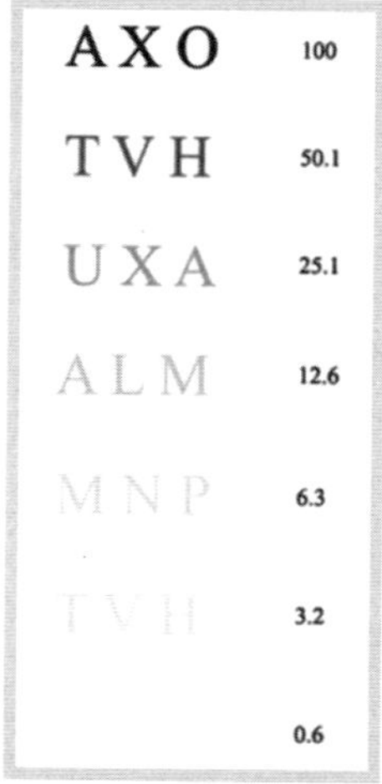

Fig. 12.33: Contrast sensitivity chart.

Testing of Contrast Sensitivity

This test measures the degree to which this ability has been lost. Large objects can be seen easily even with low contrast sensitivity but smaller objects can be seen only if contrast is of high degree.

Clinical Significance

A patient with good visual acuity but low contrast sensitivity may be suffering from diabetic retinopathy. Similarly a difference of contrast sensitivity between two eyes should be seen seriously.

COLOR VISION (FIGS. 12.34A AND B)

There are two types of photoreceptors in retina namely rods and cones. Rods work in dim light and are distributed more in peripheral

Carrier female
XX^C
X X^C
Normal male
XY
X Y
XX Normal female
X^CX Carrier female
XY Normal male
X^CY Color blind male
A

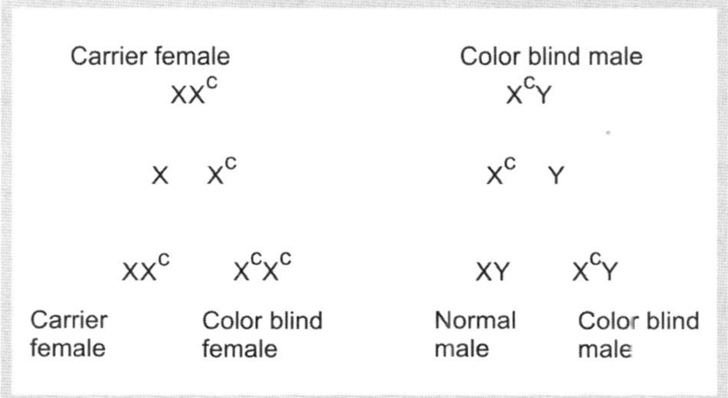

Figs. 12.34A and B: Inheritance of color vision defect.

retina. Cones work in bright light and are distributed more in macular area. Cones are also responsible for color vision. According to Young Helmholtz theory color vision is trichromatic, i.e., it is combination of three primary colors namely red, blue and green. All other colors can be made by combination of these three colors. There are three different pigments in our retina which perceive these colors. A person who cannot perceive colors properly is said to be partially color blind and another one who cannot see colors at all is said to be totally color blind. A person who is totally color blind perceives all colors as grey. This is known as Purkinje shift. Colorblindness is of two types namely **congenital** and **acquired**.

Congenital Color Blindness

It is transmitted from parents to children and till today has got no cure **(Figs. 12.34A and B)**. Males are more commonly affected (3–4%) than females (0.4%). It may be of different types:

Anomalous trichromatic color vision: Patient can appreciate all the three primary colors but one or two colors cannot be appreciated without some error. It may be of three types:
1. **Protanomalous:** Here red color perception is defective.
2. **Deuteranomalous:** Here green color perception is defective.
3. **Tritanomlous:** Here blue color perception is defective.

Dichromatic color vision: Mechanism to perceive one of the three primary colors is totally absent. Only two colors can be perceived. It may be of three types:
1. **Protanopia:** Here red color perception is absent.
2. **Deuteranopia:** Here green color perception is absent.
3. **Tritanopia:** Here blue color perception is absent.

Monochromatic color vision: Only one of the three primary colors can be appreciated. It is a very rare condition.
Achromatic color vision: It is an extremely rare condition due to congenital absence of cones. It is associated with day blindness and nystagmus. Patient is totally color blind.

Acquired Color Blindness

Due to damage to macula or optic nerve red green discrimination becomes defective. In nuclear sclerosis, blue color appreciation

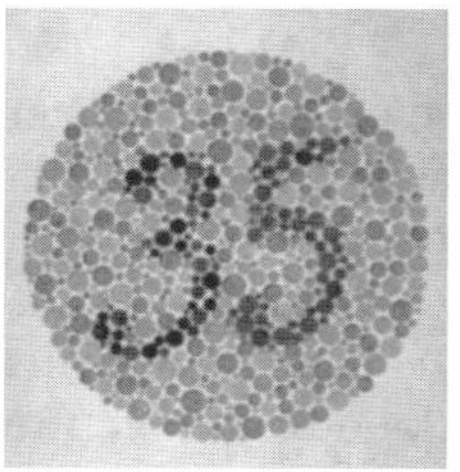
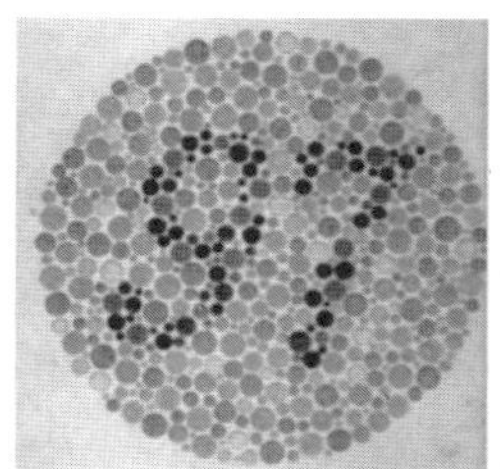
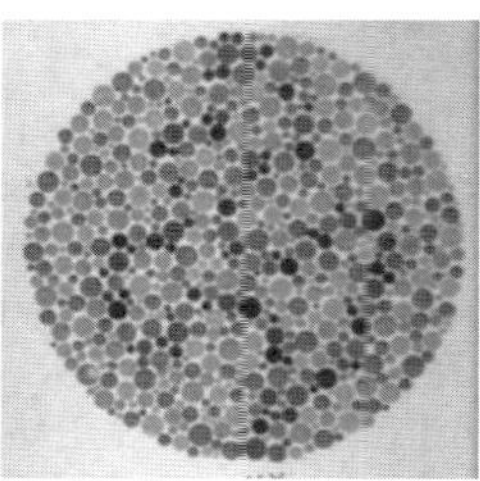

Fig. 12.35: Ishihara charts (*For color version, see Plate 2*).

becomes defective. It is because increased levels of amber color pigment in nucleus absorbs blue color.

Methods of Color Vision Testing

- Pseudoisochromatic plates, e.g., Ishihara charts **(Fig. 12.35)**
- Farnsworth Munsell 100 hue test
- City University color vision test
- Edridge green lantern test
- Nagel's anomaloscope
- Holmgren wool test

ULTRASOUND BIOMICROSCOPY

Ultrasound biomicroscopy (UBM) is a technique used to analyze anterior segment with the help of a high frequency ultrasound transducer. It is performed with a 50 MHz probe. It gives a resolution of 40 micron and a depth of 4 mm. The first commercially available machine was developed by Zeiss in 1991. The machine has three essential components:

1. Transducer
2. High frequency signal processing
3. Motion control

Transducer has a piezoelectric crystal which produces a radio-frequency pulse of 50 MHz. This radiofrequency travels the body tissues and is reflected back to the transducer. The reflected radio frequency is processed by signal processing unit and the signals are displayed on the monitor. There is a motion control device which is meant to ensure subtle movements of transducer during the procedure.

Technique

UBM is done in supine position with the eyes open. The transducer cannot come in direct contact with the cornea as there is a special cup between the eyelids to keep them open. The eyecup is filled with normal saline or sterile methylcellulose. There is approximately a distance of 2 mm between the cornea and the transducer. It prevents injury to cornea. Eyeball is scanned in each clock hour from centre of cornea to oraserrata. Images produced by UBM have a resolution of 40 microns, hence, each and every detail of different structures of anterior segment is visible.

Uses

- It helps to study angle details even in the presence of opaque medium.
- It is helpful in the study of uveitis. Presence of pars planitis, supraciliary effusion, cyclitic membrane can be seen on UBM.
- In case of trauma with hyphema, it helps to study the status of iris, lens, ciliary body, etc.
- It helps study anatomy of anterior segment in case of dense corneal opacity so that surgical intervention can be planned.
- It helps study entire extent of tumor of anterior segment.
- It helps differentiate between scleritis and episcleritis.

Limitations

- It cannot visualize structures beyond 4 mm of depth.
- UBM cannot be performed in the presence of an open corneal or sclera wound.

STERILIZATION AND DISINFECTION

Sterilization is a process which kills or removes all types of living microorganisms including bacterial spores from an article, surface or medium.

Disinfection is a process which kills or removes all types of disease causing organisms but does not kill bacterial spores.

Sterilization of Instruments

Different methods of sterilization of instruments have been depicted in the (**Flowchart 12.1**). These are:

Flowchart 12.1: Methods of sterilization.

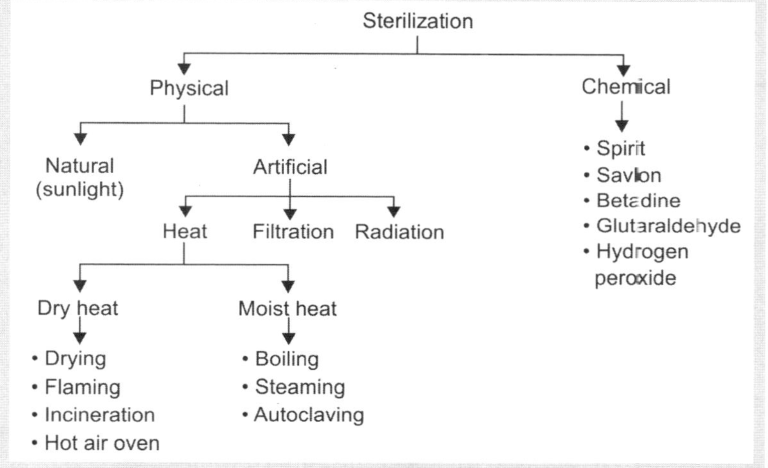

1. **Physical methods:** These may be natural like sunlight and artificial like drying, heat, filtration and radiation, etc.
2. **Chemical methods** like use of phenol, gases, halogen compounds, etc.

Sunlight is the natural method of sterilization. It contains ultraviolet rays which have lethal action against all types of microorganisms. Water in lakes, rivers and tanks are sterilized by this natural method.

Some more commonly employed methods of sterilization are:

Heat sterilization: It can be both dry and moist. Dry heat causes dehydration of cells, denaturation of proteins and oxidative damage to cells. Moist heat causes denaturation and coagulation of proteins.

Ways of Dry Heat Sterilization

- Drying in air causes dehydration of bacteria but it is an unreliable method and is of academic interest only.
- **Flaming:** Tips of forceps, hypodermic needles, scraping spatulas and tips of AC cannula can be sterilized by this method. The instrument is made red hot by keeping on the flame of a spirit lamp and allowed to cool before reusing. It kills all types of organisms including spores. Any organic material sticking to the tip should be

cleaned properly before exposing to flame. However the sharpness of the instrument is blunted.

- **Incineration:** It is used to destroy soiled dressings, blood stained cotton, beddings and pathological material.
- **Hot air oven:** It is used for forceps, scalpels, glass syringes, scissors, etc. The article must be double wrapped and kept at 150°C temperature for 2 hours.

Ways of Moist Heat Sterilization

- **Boiling:** This method kills all organisms but spores. All types of instruments can be boiled except rubber and plastic materials. Sharpness is blunted by boiling. Boiling is done for 30 minutes. Hard water should not be used as it leaves a layer of residues on all instruments and the container.
- **Steaming:** Almost all types of instruments can be steamed. It also does not kill spores. Instruments are kept over a shelf above water level and are sterilized by steaming for 30 minutes.
- **Autoclaving:** It is the best and most common method employed to sterilize all types of metallic instruments. It kills all types of micro-organisms and spores. It is done at 121°C temperature, 15 lb/inch square pressure for 20 minutes.

Sterilization Control

Spores of *Bacillus stearothermophilus* are enclosed in an envelope and kept in autoclave. Once the process of sterilization is over, these spores are inoculated on suitable medium and checked for any growth.

Chemical Sterilization is Done by Different Ways

- **Savlon:** It is composed of cetrimide and chlorhexidine. It is a surface active agent. It is effective against Gram +ve bacteria and is used to sterilize various instruments, catheters, knives and scissors, etc. It is also used for cleaning of skin for dressing.
- **Spirit:** 95% Alcohol: It does not kill viruses but is effective against bacteria and spores.
- **Methylated spirit:** It is 70% isopropyl alcohol. It is used to sterilize Schiotz tonometer.
- **Formaldehyde:** 10% formalin is used to sterilize cryoprobes, and heat sensitive instruments. Formaldehyde gas is very toxic and irritant and is used to sterilize sick rooms, wards and OT.

- **Glutaraldehyde:** It is commercially available as 'Cidex' solution and is widely used to sterilize endoscopes, rubber tubings, catheters. It is very effective against tubercle bacilli, fungi and viruses.
- **Hydrogen peroxide:** 3% solution is very effective against HIV and Herpes. It is commonly used to clean dirty wounds, prisms, lenses and applanation tonometers
- **Ethylene oxide gas:** It is used to sterilize IOLs, DCR tubings, disposable plastic items like catheters, syringes, etc. It is very effective against bacteria, spores and viruses.

Sterilization by Radiation

X-rays, Gamma rays, cosmic rays are ionizing radiations. They are lethal to DNA and kill all types of microorganisms. They penetrate tissues without raising the temperature. They are used to sterilize plastic items like syringes, catheters, etc.

Infrared rays are nonionizing radiations. They are absorbed by the surface and temperature of the article is raised. They are used for rapid mass sterilization of syringes, and hospital wards, virus laboratories, etc.

Sterilization of Operation Theater

The process of sterilization of operation theater (OT) is known as *fumigation*.

First of all OT is cleaned nicely and washed with soap and water thoroughly. All the walls should be thoroughly mopped. Once the room has been air dried, it is fumigated with formalin solution.

Availability of Formalin

Formalin is commercially available as 40% solution. When it is heated vapors of formaldehyde are produced. It is best done at 20°C temperature and 65% of relative humidity. The quantity of 40% formalin required is 0.50 mL per cubic foot.

For an area of 1,000 cubic foot 500 mL of 40% formalin solution is added in 1,000 mL of water in an electric boiler. Boiler is switched on after sealing the door. After about one hour when whole of the solution has vaporized, the boiler is switched off from outside the OT.

Formaldehyde vapors can also be produced by automatic vaporizing unit operated electrically.

Alternatively for 1,000 cubic foot area of OT, 450 g of potassium permanganate is added to 500 mL of 40% formalin solution. This causes auto-boiling and generates fumes. This is an exothermic reaction and takes place vigorously hence must be carried out by an expert technician.

OT is closed for 24–48 hours. After opening the OT after 48 hours, AC is turned on and residual vapors are allowed to escape in a proper way so that there is no problem with the other hospital staff. To neutralize the residual formalin 150 mL of 10% ammonia is taken in a bowl for 500 mL of formalin used and kept in the centre of the OT for three hours.

Example: For an OT of 20 × 15 × 10 size = 3,000 cubic foot area, 1,500 mL of 40% formalin will be required for fumigation and 450 mL of 10% ammonia will be required for neutralization of residual fumes.

Procedure

Seal all the possible outlets of OT through which formaldehyde gas can leak. Place spore strips in OT at appropriate places to check decontamination. Place the vaporizing unit in the room and close the door from outside. Seal this door from outside. Put the unit on and wait for about one hour till whole of the solution is used up. The OT is kept locked till 24 hours. After 24 hours, the air conditioner is put on, the door is opened and the gas is allowed to leak out in a proper way. Nobody is allowed to enter the room till the gas has been allowed to escape. Levels of residual gas are checked with a suitable air monitoring equipment. It should be as low as 2 ppm. Formaldehyde gas is a scheduled chemical and is very harmful for humans. Its maximum exposure limit is 2 ppm. Thus the fumigation must be carried out by a trained paramedical staff as per the described procedure.

Caution: *Hydrochloric acid and chlorine containing compounds must not be present in OT as formaldehyde gas can react with these compounds to form a lung carcinogen (Chloromethyl).*

Lasers in Ophthalmology

LASER stands for *Light Amplification for Stimulated Emission of Radiation*. There are different types of clinical applications of different types of laser systems. Commonly employed procedures are:

YAG CAPSULOTOMY

YAG stands for 'Yttrium Aluminium Garnet'. This type of solid state laser is used for treatment of 'After Cataract'. After extracapsular cataract extraction (ECCE) or small incision cataract surgery (SCIS) or phacoemulsification posterior capsule becomes thick and opaque. Patient starts complaining of blurring of vision. On slit lamp examination with dilated pupil thick posterior capsule can be easily appreciated. With the help of YAG laser a hole is made in the posterior capsule in front of pupil. It is an OPD procedure and patient is sent home immediately after the procedure. Usually, 1.6 to 3.2 mJ of energy is required to make a hole of 2 to 3 mm just opposite the pupil. 2 to 4 shots are sufficient to serve the purpose. Too big or too small holes should be avoided to prevent cystoids macular edema (CME).

YAG IRIDOTOMY

In patients who are prone to develop narrow angle glaucoma peripheral iridotomy can be done by using YAG laser to prevent attack of acute congestive glaucoma **(Fig. 13.1)**.

LASER FOR PHOTOCOAGULATION IN RETINAL DISORDERS

Neovascularization of retina, e.g., in diabetes, Eales' disease, branch retinal vein occlusion (BRVO), branch retinal artery occlusion (BRAO), etc., can be taken care of by photocoagulation otherwise it can cause vitreous hemorrhage or neovascular glaucoma

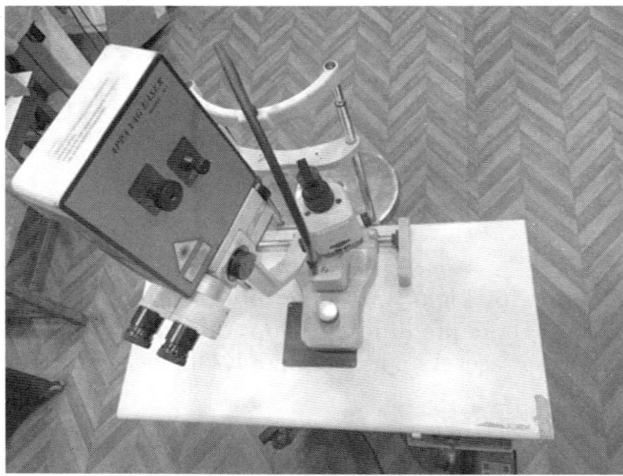

Fig. 13.1: YAG laser.

leading to blindness. Here argon laser or diode laser is used. The purpose of laser is to decrease the oxygen demand of retina. The part of retina which is lasered becomes dead, hence, no oxygen is required by that part. At the same time that part of retina becomes nonseeing. Macular area and hence, central vision is spared in this procedure so that patient can see and carry out his routine activities **(Figs. 13.2 and 13.3)**.

EXCIMER LASER AND LASIK LASER FOR CORNEAL REFRACTIVE SURGERY

This surgery is used widely nowaday to get rid of spectacles. In photorefractive keratectomy (PRK) epithelium of cornea is abraded, excimer laser is applied on the bed, soft bandage contact lens is put and patient is sent home with the advice to come back after five days when all the epithelium is regenerated and there is no refractive error left. In C-LASIK laser and SBK (Sub-Bowman's keratomileusis or tissue saving profile) a flap of cornea is raised with a microkeratome, excimer laser is applied on the bed, flap put in its position and patient is allowed to go home. Advantage of this type of laser over excimer laser C Lasik and SBK over PRK is that the patient does not complain of pain, redness, etc., because epithelium remains intact. This laser

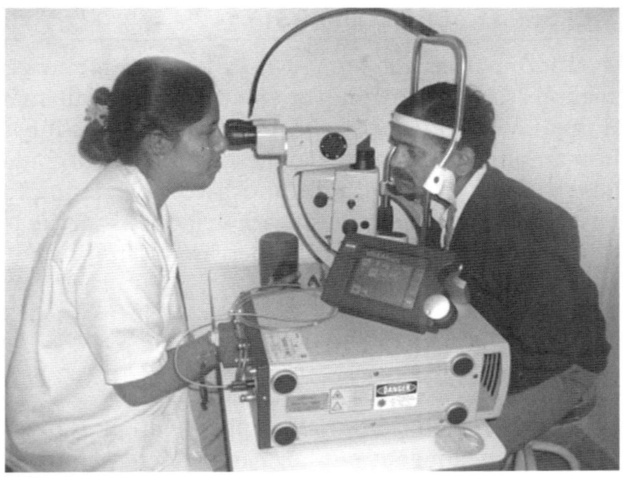

Fig. 13.2: Laser for retinal photocoagulation.

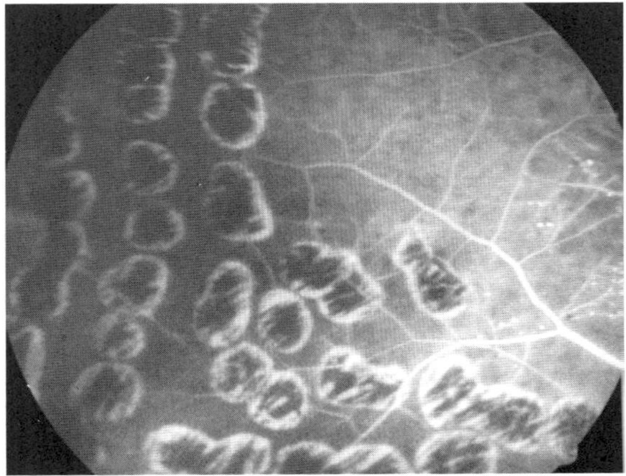

Fig. 13.3: Laser spots on retina.

uses argon fluoride gas as substrate for producing laser beam and hence is called a gas state laser.

4.Nd:Glass (Femtosecond) Lasers: This laser is being used to create corneal flaps in Z LASIK or femtosecond LASIK. It is also used in small incision lenticule extraction (SMILE) and smooth incision lenticule keratomileusis (SILK) surgeries to get rid of spectacles.

ARGON LASER TRABECULOPLASTY

Patients suffering from glaucoma who are not fit for surgery and intraocular pressure (IOP) cannot be controlled even with maximum medical therapy, argon laser trabeculoplasty (ALT) is the answer. Laser shots are applied on trabecular meshwork through gonioscope. This causes localized burning of meshwork. Scarring follows, which has a pulling effect on meshwork that opens up the pores of trabeculum, thus aqueous outflow is increased. This procedure can control rise in IOP for a couple of years.

ROLE OF LASER IN TRABECULECTOMY (UNDER-FILTERING BLEB)

After this surgery if bleb is not well formed and IOP is high due to underfiltering bleb, aqueous outflow can be increased by breaking one of the sutures with the help of laser.

LASER IN TREATMENT OF MALIGNANT GLAUCOMA

In this glaucoma aqueous pockets are formed in the vitreous cavity due to misdirection of aqueous humor. Specific treatment consists of breaking vitreous phase with the help of laser and letting the aqueous humor come out of these pockets.

LASER FOR DCR SURGERY

Endolaser dacryocystorhinostomy (DCR) is gaining popularity nowaday as this procedure does not require any incision, so it is more acceptable cosmetically as compared to conventional DCR.

14

CHAPTER

Contact Lens Practice

A contact lens is a small plastic wafer designed to rest on cornea or sclera and is used to correct refractive errors. It may be of three types **(Fig. 14.1)**:

1. Soft contact lens
2. Semisoft contact lens
3. Hard contact lens

NOMENCLATURE

- **Overall diameter:** The dimension across the physical boundary of contact lens in millimeter. It may be 13 mm, 13.5 mm or 14 mm in case soft contact lens. It varies according to size of cornea and type of lens. Overall diameter of semisoft contact lens is smaller than overall diameter of soft contact lens.
- **Optic zone:** It is the central part of contact lens used to focus rays of light on retina. It is decided as per size of pupil and overall diameter.
- **Base curve:** It is the curvature of posterior central part of contact lens which rests on anterior surface of cornea. It is decided by K.
- **Peripheral curves:** These are 2–3 depending on make of lens and help to stabilize contact lens on cornea.
- **Edge:** It is union of anterior and posterior curves at the periphery.
- **Power:** It is decided by anterior central curvature of contact lens and varies according to refractive error of patient.
- **Thickness:** It is measured at the central part of lens in millimeter.
- **Tint:** It is the color of lens.
- K refers to the flatter of the two meridians of cornea (higher reading of keratometry in millimeter) **(Fig. 14.2)**.

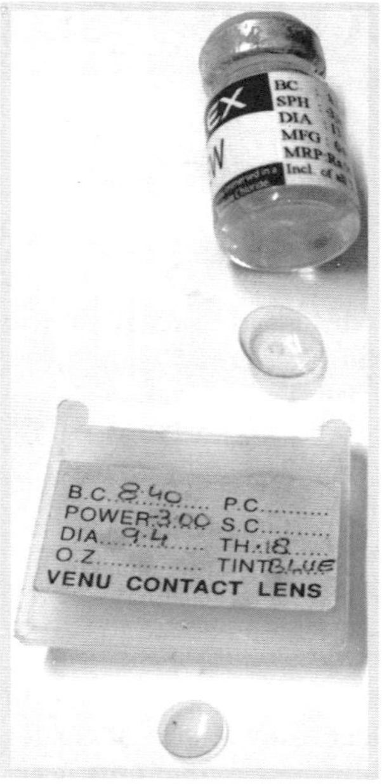

Fig. 14.1: Soft and semisoft contact lens.

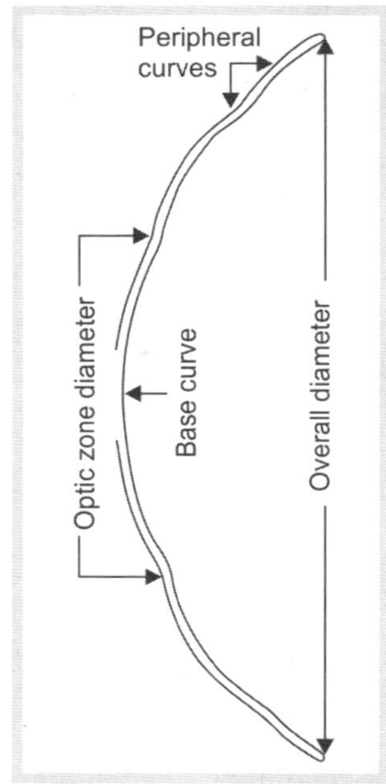

Fig. 14.2: Parts of contact lens.

ANATOMY AND PHYSIOLOGY OF CORNEA

Cornea is transparent, avascular structure present on anterior surface of eyeball. Its diameter on anterior surface is 11.7 mm horizontally and 11 mm vertically. Its thickness is 0.54 mm in center and power is +45 D. Radius of curvature is 7.94 mm. It has got five layers **(Fig. 14.3)**:

1. **Epithelium:** It is the most anterior, metabolically most active layer of cornea. It is made up of many layers of cells. Each cell is richly supplied with nerves from ophthalmic branch of trigeminal nerve. Thus it causes pain when a cell is damaged. It has a very good repair capacity.
2. **Bowman's membrane:** This is the layer which does not have regenerative capacity. Damage to this layer may leave corneal opacity.
3. **Stroma or substantia propria:** It constitutes 90% thickness of cornea. It is made up of multilayered lamellae. Metabolically, it is less active. Its peculiar arrangement makes the cornea transparent.

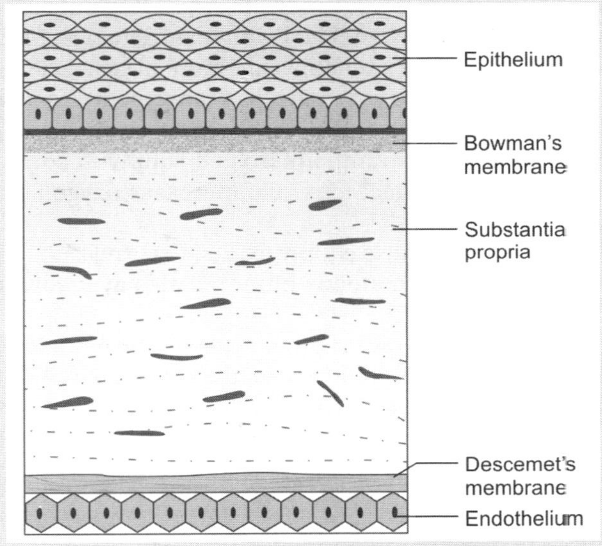

Fig. 14.3: Microscopic structure of cornea.

4. **Descemet's membrane:** It is very resilient and does not give way easily.
5. **Endothelium:** It is second most active layer of cornea. It has hexagonal cells, each cell has sodium potassium ATPase pump which keeps on pushing water out of cornea that enters its substance and keeps it transparent. Any damage to these cells is repaired by enlargement of neighboring cells. Normal endothelial cell count is 3000/mm^3 . Damage to this layer results in loss of transparency. Cell count decreases with age. Cornea decompensates if cell count decreases less than 300/mm^3.

Oxygen Supply of Cornea

Cornea gets oxygen in different ways:

- Most important source is atmospheric oxygen dissolved in tears (precorneal tear film). When a person wears contact lenses, this supply of oxygen is decreased. Now the supply depends on two factors. Firstly, the material that may or may not allow oxygen to pass through its substance. This depends on DK value of the material. Higher is the DK value, more oxygen can pass through the substance of cornea. Secondly, the movement of contact lens on cornea that is directly related with tear exchange. More is the blink rate, more is tear exchange and more oxygen is available to cornea. Steep (tight) fitting causes less movement of contact lens, thus less tear exchange and lesser oxygen is available to cornea. Thick contact lens also impairs oxygen supply to cornea. High water content of contact lens also increases oxygen supply to cornea.

- Perilimbal capillaries also supply oxygen to cornea.
- Oxygen dissolved in aqueous humor is also available to inner layers of cornea.

During sleep oxygen supply to cornea is decreased remarkably. If we sleep with contact lens on our cornea, the oxygen supply is further decreased leading to corneal hypoxia. Cornea becomes edematous, with microcysts. Eyes become red and person may complain of blurring of vision. Thus it is strongly recommended that one must not sleep with contact lens on cornea.

PRECORNEAL TEAR FILM

A very thin layer of tears covers the cornea known as precorneal tear film. It has three layers **(Fig. 14.4)**:

1. **Mucin layer:** It is secreted by mucin secretory glands of conjunctiva namely goblet cells, crypts of Henle and glands of Manz. It converts hydrophobic surface of cornea into hydrophilic surface thus stabilizing the aqueous layer of tear film on cornea.
2. **Aqueous layer:** It constitutes main bulk of tear film. It is secreted by accessory lacrimal glands namely glands of Krause and glands of Wolfring. It forms the basic tear secretion. The main lacrimal gland secrets tears during hours of emotional crisis known as reflex tear secretion. This layer keeps the cornea and conjunctiva moist, flushes away the metabolic waste products from conjunctiva. This layer contains sodium chloride, sugar, and urea. It is alkaline in nature and saltish to taste. It also contains antibacterial substances like lysozyme, betalysin and lactoferrin.
3. **Lipid layer:** It is secreted by meibomian glands. It spreads over the aqueous layer and prevents its evaporation. It also lubricates the eyelids to facilitate blinking.

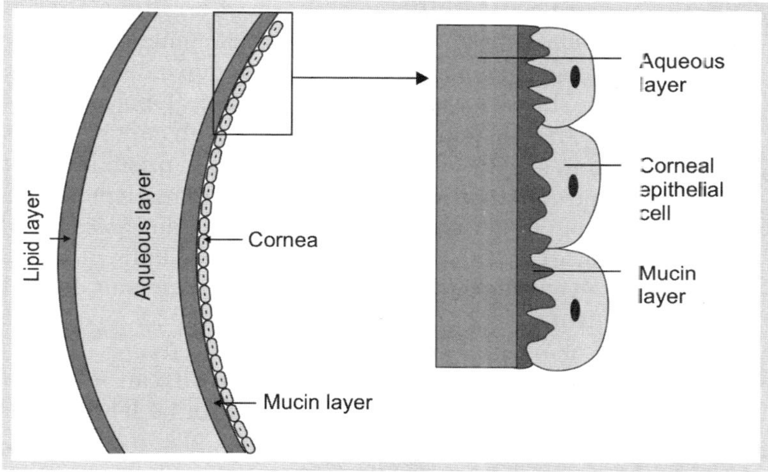

Fig. 14.4: Precorneal tear film.

Functions of Tear Film

- It supplies oxygen to cornea.
- It keeps the cornea and conjunctiva moist.
- It contains antibacterial substances.
- It flushes away the metabolic waste products from conjunctiva and cornea.
- It facilitates blinking. Normal blink rate is 12 per minute.

Tear production is decreased in old age, during hours of fatigue. Use of certain drugs like timolol, pilocarpine, oral contraceptives, antihistaminics decreases tear production. Thus such medicines should not be used by a contact lens wearer. Pregnancy also decreases tear production.

INDICATIONS AND CONTRAINDICATIONS OF CONTACT LENS

Contact lenses can be used for different purposes such as:

- **Optical indications:** Myopia, hypermetropia, astigmatism, keratoconus (cone-shaped cornea), anisometropia and aniseikonia, aphakia, presbyopia, aniridia (absence of iris) and albinism (absence of melanin pigment). Refractive errors are better corrected with contact lenses as compared to spectacles because of larger field, little peripheral aberrations and no rim interference. It has been found that axial length is slightly decreased by using contact lenses in myopia due to its flattening effect. Thus it slows down progress of myopia. Hypermetropes exert less accommodation and convergence with contact lenses as compared to spectacles. It is due to base out prism effect of spectacles during convergence. Irregular astigmatism can be corrected by contact lenses only. In anisometropia and aniseikonia spectacles cause disparity of image size leading to diplopia. These conditions can be rectified by using contact lenses. In aniridia and albinism patient cannot tolerate light (photophobia). A cosmetic contact lens can be used to avoid photophobia.

- **Cosmetic indications:** Unsightly cornea or eyeballs can be hidden by tinted or painted contact lenses. Pupil can be left clear in contact lens if eye has got some useful vision. Color of underlying iris can be changed by cosmetic contact lens as is required by some actors.
- **Occupational indications:** Sports persons get an advantage of getting less serious injury with contact lens. News casters and television actors can avoid reflections by using contact lens. Fogging of spectacles can be avoided while shifting from cold or hot and humid atmosphere.
- **Therapeutic indications:** Soft contact lenses have been found useful in treatment of nonhealing corneal ulcers, impending corneal perforation, bullous keratopathy, trichiasis, prevention of symblepharon, recurrent corneal erosions, etc. Medicines like pilocarpine have been found more effective when they are instilled over contact lens or incorporated in contact lens.
- **Diagnostic indications:** Procedures such as gonioscopy, fundoscopy and electrodiagnostic procedures like ERG are done taking help of contact lens.
- **Research indications:** Contact lenses can be used for research purposes like occlusion of eye in animals, stimulating accommodation and relaxing accommodation.

Contraindications of Contact Lens

- **Infective conditions of eye:** Stye, chalazion, blepharitis, conjunctivitis, keratitis, etc. Use of contact lens in such circumstances can spread infection.

- Allergic eye conditions like spring catarrh, simple allergic conjunctivitis. Symptoms may be exaggerated.
- Abnormalities of lid margin like entropion and ectropion, trichiasis and diseases of conjunctiva like pterygium, limbal dermoid (due to surface irregularity fitting is not proper).
- Paralysis of fifth nerve causes loss of corneal sensations and contact lens can damage the cornea without awareness of the patient.
- Exophthalmos causes improper blinking and tear exchange becomes inadequate.
- Ocular conditions like scleritis, episcleritis, uveitis, bleb of trabeculectomy, uncontrolled diabetes.
- **Nonmedical conditions:** If patient is not motivated failure is likely to occur. Failures are more in males than females, hypermetropes than myopes, high astigmatism, better vision with glasses and patients with large pupils.
- **Tear film disturbances:** Contact lenses themselves cause dry eye, so should not be used in dry eye conditions.

MATERIALS USED FOR MANUFACTURING OF CONTACT LENS

Different materials used for manufacturing of contact lenses are:

- **Polymethyl methacrylate (PMMA):** PMMA has good optical properties, inert, nontoxic having excellent moulding and machining qualities but practically impermeable to oxygen. Thus the lenses made from it can be used only for a limited time. It has transmission of 90%, ref. index of 1.49, hardness of 4.5 as compared to 10 of diamond. Its softness makes it vulnerable to scratches. It has 1.5% water content after immersion in solution for several days. A thin coating of silicon tetrachloride increases its wettability.
- **Polycarbonate:** It is transparent, tough with high refractive index, more prone to scratching than PMMA. It is used for high power contact lenses.
- **Cellulose acetate butyrate (CAB):** It is hard, strong with good machining and moulding properties.
- **Silicone rubber:** It is also a good material. However, it is hydrophobic in nature and a hydrophilic coating needs to be done on the surface of contact lens.

- **Hexa Ethyl Meth Acrylate (HEMA):** HEMA and its copolymers are commonly used to make soft contact lenses.
- **Fluorocarbons:** These are newer materials with very good oxygen permeability.

Properties of Contact Lens Material

Materials used in manufacturing of contact lens should have following properties:

- It should be biologically inert, i.e., it should not react with tissues it comes in contact with.
- It should have high gas permeability.
- It should have little friction effect between contact lens and eye tissues.
- It should not change its properties when subjected to different pH.
- It should not take part in enzymatic activities.
- It should not absorb metabolites and toxins.
- It should not show strong adhesive molecular forces.
- It should not show excessive electrophoretic osmotic properties.
- It should not excite inflammatory response even if it remains in contact with the tissue over a long duration of time.

PARAMETERS OF CONTACT LENS

- **Power:** It is determined by curvature of anterior surface of optic zone of contact lens. It is not related directly with thickness of lens. It is calculated by doing refraction and taking help of conversion table.
- **Base curve:** It is decided by curvature of anterior surface of cornea as determined by keratometry. Base curve of soft contact lens is made flatter than flat K of cornea because the overall diameter of soft contact lens is always greater than greatest diameter of cornea. However, diameter of semisoft/hard contact lens is smaller than diameter of cornea so its base curve is kept same as flat K of cornea.
- **Overall diameter:** It depends upon diameter of cornea which can be taken either by a caliper or a simple scale.
- **Thickness:** More is the thickness of lens lesser will be the oxygen permeability. In addition it makes the lens heavier and it tends to fall thus making the fit flatter. Most of the manufacturing companies keep this parameter of contact lens constant.

- **Optic zone diameter:** It is usually kept constant, however, it can be increased or decreased depending upon size of pupil.
- **Edges:** They should be smooth.
- **Water content:** More is the water content, more is the oxygen permeability so that person can wear the contact lens for a longer duration. However, it becomes thicker, heavier and more pliable with increasing water content. Accordingly, parameters have to be set to have alignment fitting.
- **Oxygen permeability:** It depends on DK value of material, thickness of lens and water content of lens. Higher DK value means more oxygen permeability. More thickness of lens means lesser oxygen permeability. High water content means higher oxygen permeability. High oxygen permeability increases wearing period of contact lens.

HISTORY TAKING FOR CONTACT LENS FITTING

- Why do you want contact lens? Whether the reason is cosmetic, optical, occupational or any other.
- Any history of ocular surgery. Contact lens should not be prescribed immediately after glaucoma surgery to avoid injury to bleb.
- History of diabetes? Whether taking any medicines? Whether blood sugar levels are within normal limits? Contact lens should not be prescribed to uncontrolled diabetics. Pregnancy can also trouble the patient who is already using contact lens due to water logging.
- History of drug intake? Drugs like antihistaminic (cetirizine, avil), oral contraceptives, decongestants, beta-blockers interfere with contact lens wear. It is advised that no drug should be used over contact lenses except preservative free lubricating eyedrops.
- History of any previous contact lens failure, if yes try to find out the cause to avoid repeated failure.
- History of ocular allergy or infection or dryness. If yes, treat the cause first.

Examination

- Vision with and without glasses and with pin hole should be recorded.

- Any evidence of disease of conjunctiva, cornea, lids, etc., like blepharitis, pterygium, vascularization of cornea, etc.
- Any evidence of dry eye.
- Any evidence of recent ocular surgery.
- Keratometry, corneal diameter, diameter of pupil, corneal sensation, tear film break-up time (BUT) and blinking.

Aircrew members are not allowed to use contact lens, however, air hostess can do so. Contact lenses are not allowed in mining, sand blasting and drilling.

FITTING OF CONTACT LENS

If patient is a beginner, she must be given a trial of contact lens. Different types of fittings are **(Figs. 14.5A to C)**:

- **Alignment fitting:** This is the ideal fitting in which contact lens floats on precorneal tear film. There is neither pooling of dye (tears) anywhere nor the contact lens touches the cornea. Movements of contact lens with each blink are sufficient enough to enable tear exchange required by cornea.
- **Steep (tight) fitting:** Here the contact lens touches the cornea at periphery and there is pooling of dye (tears) at the center of cornea. Contact lens shows very little movement with each blink

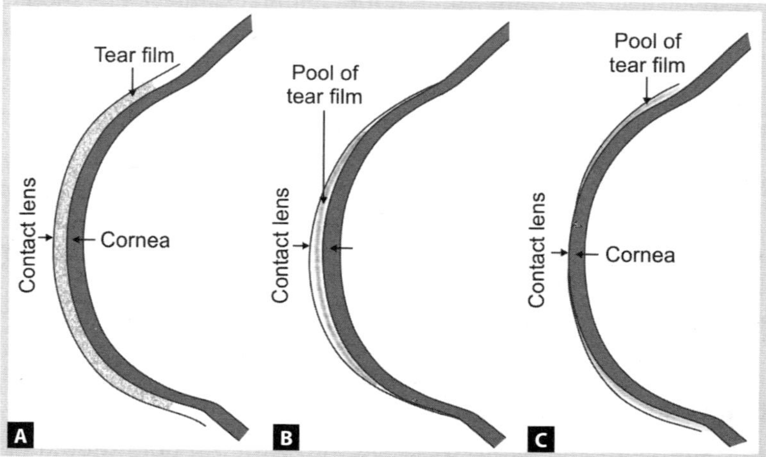

Figs. 14.5A to C: Types of fitting. (A) Alignment fit; (B) Steep fit; (C) Flat fit.

so that tear exchange is inadequate and cornea is at risk of hypoxia (lack of oxygen supply). However, due to very little movement patient feels quite comfortable immediately after wearing contact lens but starts having problem after some time due to hypoxia. Steep fitting is dangerous and should be avoided.

- **Flat (loose) fitting:** Here the contact lens touches the cornea at center and there is pooling of tears at the periphery. Movements of contact lens on cornea are more than normal. There is adequate tear exchange and no risk of hypoxia at all. However, excessive movements of contact lens give foreign body sensation and patient feels uncomfortable and takes more time to adjust with lenses.

How to Start Contact Lens Fitting?

- Find power of contact lens by doing refraction. Power of spectacles needs to be converted into power of contact lens by consulting conversion table. Power of cylinder needs to be made half (called spherical equivalent) and added algebraically to power of sphere, e.g., if power of spectacles is +1.00 DS, +2.00 DS, +3.00 DS or –1.00 DS, –2.00 DS, –3.00 DS; the power of contact lens will remain same. If power of spectacles is +4.00 DS, +10.00 DS; power of contact lens needs to be increased. If power of spectacles is –5.00 DS, –8.00 DS; power of contact lens needs to be decreased as is evident from the **Table 14.1**.
  If power of spectacles is –4.00 DS/–1.00 DC × 180°, the power of contact lens will be (–3.75 DS) + (–0.50 DS) {spherical equivalent of cylinder} = –4.25 DS.
- Base curve of contact lens is calculated by doing keratometry and adding 0.70 to flat K reading (for soft contact lens), e.g., if K readings are 7.80 and 7.90, base curve of soft contact lens will be 7.90 + 0.70 = 8.60. Base curve of semisoft contact lens is taken as flat K reading, i.e., 7.90.
- Diameter of contact lens is calculated by adding 2.00 to greatest diameter of cornea measured by scale or caliper for soft contact lens and by deducing 2.00 from minimum diameter of cornea for semisoft contact lens. However, every manufacturer keeps diameter of its make fairly constant and alignment fitting is achieved by changing base curve.
- Tint of contact lens and its water content can be decided in consultation with the patient.

Table 14.1: Conversion table.

Sl. No.	Power of spectacles (DS)	Power of CL (DS)	Power of spectacles (DS)	Power of CL (DS)
1.	+1.00	+1.00	–1.00	–1.00
2.	+2.00	+2.00	–2.00	–2.00
3.	+3.00	+3.00	–3.00	–3.00
4.	+4.00	+4.25	–4.00	–3.75
5.	+5.00	+5.50	–5.00	–4.50
6.	+6.00	+6.75	–6.00	–5.50
7.	+7.00	+7.75	–7.00	–6.25
8.	+8.00	+9.00	–8.00	–7.00
9.	+9.00	+10.25	–9.00	–7.75
10.	+10.00	+11.75	–10.00	–8.75
11.	+12.00	+14.50	–12.00	–10.00
12.	+14.00	+17.75	–14.00	–11.50
13.	+16.00	+21.00	–16.00	–13.00

HOW TO INSERT SOFT CONTACT LENS?

There are different ways of inserting soft contact lens (CL): Wet the tip of right index finger. Put soft contact lens on finger tip. Pull the upper eyelid of right eye with other hand and lower eyelid with middle finger of right hand. Put contact lens by looking directly onto the contact lens.

Fitting Technique

- Ask the patient to wash her hands and eyes with soap and water. Shake excess water.
- Take contact lens and check inside out and right left.
- Wet contact lens should be put on finger and introduced in the eye. Ask the patient to move her eyeball so that the lens settles on cornea.
- If patient experiences foreign body sensation ask her to close the eyes for 15–30 minutes.
- Do slit-lamp examination for type of fitting. Base curve of contact lens or diameter of contact lens can be adjusted to achieve alignment fitting. Following points should be looked for:

- **Centration:** Contact lens should be nicely centered on cornea. Cornea should be properly covered by contact lens.
- **Movements of contact lens:** With each blink contact lens should move 0.5–1.00 mm, lesser movements indicate steep fit and greater movements indicate flat fit.

- In semisoft and hard contact lens fitting, fluorescein stain is used. By this method pooling of dye (green area) and corneal touch (blue area) can be easily appreciated.

Fluorescein stain is never used in soft contact lens fitting as the soft contact lenses absorb dye and become unfit for use.

Advantages of Semisoft Contact Lens Over Soft Contact Lens

- Visual acuity is better with semisoft contact lens.
- High astigmatism can be corrected better with semisoft contact lens.
- Irregular astigmatism and keratoconus can be corrected only with semisoft contact lens.
- Semisoft contact lens can be worn for a longer duration as compared to soft contact lens.
- Oxygen supply to cornea is much better with semisoft contact lens.
- They are more durable and require lesser care.
- Modification can be done in semisoft contact lens after manufacturing but it is not possible in soft contact lens.

However, their fitting technique needs to be mastered. They take more time for adaptation because their edge rests on cornea (very sensitive) while in soft contact lens the edge rests on sclera (less sensitive).

INSTRUCTIONS TO THE PATIENT

Always:

- Wash your hands before inserting or removing CL.
- Clean CL after removing and before inserting.
- Store them in CL solution.
- Wear CL according to wearing schedule.
- Carry your specs and CL kit with you while traveling.
- Cosmetics (Kajal, Surma) should be applied after putting the lens.

- Perfumes should be sprayed well before putting the CL because these are alcohol based chemicals and remain in air as aerosols for some time. They are absorbed by contact lens, which can damage the cornea.

Never:

- Wet your CL by placing in mouth.
- Rub your CL with tissue paper.
- Sleep with CL on. One can have a nap.
- Wash your CL in tap water. It can cause infection of acanthamoeba.
- Put them in hot water. They can get warped.
- Insert over a sink. Many lenses are lost down the drain.
- To begin with CL should be used for a short period. Wearing period can be increased gradually.

CLEANING OF LENSES

Contact lenses should be cleaned after and before every use. Deproteinization of lenses should be done every 15 days. Protein content of tears gets deposited on contact lens due to opposite charge and alters the optical quality of contact lens. Contact lens should be placed in a clean vial along with CL solution and an enzyme tablet. The vial should be closed and kept for 4–6 hours. Protein deposits are dissolved by action of enzyme. CL is taken out and the CL solution of vial is discarded. After cleaning with fresh CL solution the contact lenses are ready for use.

Disinfection of Contact Lens

There are two ways of disinfection:

1. **Thermal:** Contact lenses must be deproteinized before disinfection. The CL should be put in a vial with CL solution and cap tightly closed. Put this whole vial in boiling water for 30 minutes. Let the water cool and CL is ready for use. This procedure can also be done with the help of Soft Lens Aseptor-Patient Unit.
2. **Chemical:** This is a less commonly employed method.

POSTFITTING PROBLEMS AND SOLUTION

- **Foreign body sensation:** Some amount of foreign body (FB) sensation is common after initial contact lens use. This is a part of adaptation. However, if this sensation lasts for long following things should be looked for:

- Excessive movements of lens
- Bad finish of edge
- A low riding lens which strikes the lower lid

Solution: Excessive movements can be appreciated on slit lamp examination. Bad finish of edge can be felt by tip of index finger. A low riding lens can be easily seen even on torch light examination. Excessive movements are due to loose/flat fit. To rectify decrease the base curve of contact lens, increase the overall diameter of contact lens or decrease the thickness of lens. A bad finish of edge can be corrected by refinishing the contact lens. A low riding lens can be rectified by steepening the base curve or increasing overall diameter or making the lens thin. Similarly an up riding lens can be rectified by increasing the overall diameter, steepening the base curve, increasing the thickness of optic zone or decreasing the thickness of periphery.

Sometimes while traveling patient complains of some foreign particle going inside the eye and creating FB sensation. Remove the lens; wash the eye with clean water. If FB sensation is no more, reinsert the lens after cleaning it with CL solution. If still the FB sensation persists, consult the nearest eye surgeon.

- **Edge in the pupil:** Patient complains of transient but frequent blurring of vision. This is due to nonoptical area of lens coming in and going out of pupillary area. This problem can be dealt by increasing the optic zone diameter of contact lens or overall diameter of contact lens and steepening the base curve if it is flat fit.

Special Types of Contact Lenses

Scleral Lenses (Fig. 14.6)

Scleral lenses are large diameter lenses which can be worn for extended period of time over anterior ocular surface. It rests on conjunctiva/sclera. It has minimal clearance between corneal portion of lens and cornea/limbus.

Advantages

Scleral lenses are of immense importance in advanced keratoconus or severe irregular corneas, patients who require high toric powers and prisms, pathological and disfigured eyes, greatly decentred pupil,

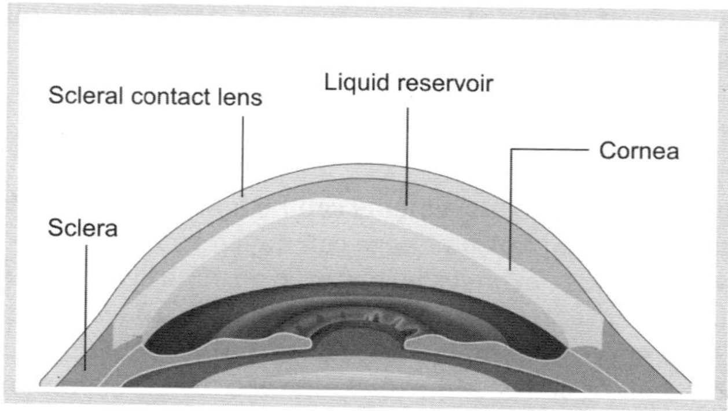

Fig. 14.6: Scleral contact lens.

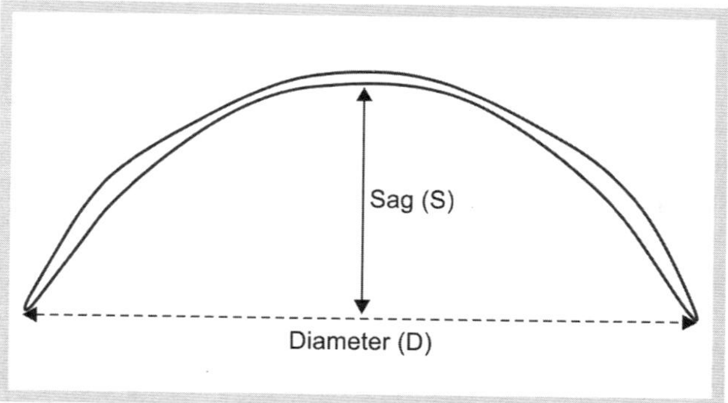

Fig. 14.7: Sag height.

patients involved in active water sports and vigorous sports because scleral CLs are more stable over cornea as compared to other types of contact lenses, post RK patients and special effects for performing arts.

There are certain disadvantages of scleral lenses like long fitting time, cost factor, limited availability and specialist required for fitting.

Types of Scleral Lenses Based on their Overall Diameter

- **Corneoscleral:** 12.9–13.5 mm
- **Semi-scleral:** 13.6–14.9 mm
- **Mini-scleral:** 15.0–18.0 mm
- **Full scleral:** 18.1–24.0 mm

There are different zones in scleral lens:

- **Optic zone:** This is the central part of scleral lens that lies in front of pupil of patient. It is meant to create desired optical effect. Base curve and dioptric power incorporated in this zone controls the sag height of the lens. **Sag height (Fig. 14.7)** is the depth of scleral lens between a tangent drawn at the center of the optic zone and an imaginary line drawn at the peripheral boundary of scleral lens.
- **Landing zone:** It is the peripheral part of scleral lens which rests on sclera and tries to mimic shape of anterior ocular surface. It is very important for providing stability to scleral lens and achieving proper alignment fit of lens. It is also referred to as the scleral or haptic zone. An adequate and even distribution of pressure over this area creates adequate corneal clearance mandatory to avoid any corneal damage during wear.
- **Transition zone:** It is also referred to as the midperipheral or **limbal zone** lying between optical zone and the landing zone. It consists of series of peripheral curves.
- **Corneal clearance zone:** Scleral lenses vault over the cornea without touching it, so that a space is left between cornea and contact lens which gets filled with tears or normal saline. This space acts as a reservoir, providing hydration and lubrication to the cornea throughout the day. This is good for corneal health.

Fitting: It is primarily based on sag height (depth of scleral lens between a tangent drawn at the center of the optic zone and an imaginary line drawn at the peripheral boundary of scleral lens), K readings are of limited use.

Step 1: Diameter—it helps to alter the amount of corneal clearance. Smaller diameter is used in cases of normal corneas whereas larger diameter becomes a better choice in cases of compromised and disfigured eyes.
Step 2: Clearance—a minimum 100 microns to 500 microns of corneal clearance is required. The measurement can be done by comparison with normal corneal thickness or contact lens thickness. Excessive clearance reduces visual acuity. Limbal clearance should be about 100 microns. Limbal staining should be monitored and avoided.

Step 3: Landing zone fit—it can show following abnormal findings:

- Flat fit-air bubbles in periphery
- Excessive bearing causes compression and leads to blanching.

Step 4: Lens edge—3 factors to be considered—scleral alignment, blanching/impingement and edge lift:

- Too much edge lift causes CL awareness and discomfort
- Low edge lift causes full/partial impingement.

Step 5: Movement—slight movement acceptable as it is better for tear exchange.

Step 6: Over-refraction—now because an irregular corneal surface has been replaced by a regular surface of scleral lens hence retinoscopy can be done and refractive error can be adjusted in the scleral lens to be ordered for this patient. This error will be incorporated in the new scleral lens itself.

Factors necessary for a good fit:

- Corneal clearance essential
- Fenestration necessary
- Adequate tear layer thickness
- Absence of bubbles, especially in pupillary area
- No perilimbal touch
- Lens tolerance, good vision and continued comfort should be the goal

Lens insertion/removal:

- Use either tripod technique using 3 fingers/plunger technique
- Make the patient sit comfortably and bend the head parallel to the ground
- Hold the lens and fill it with saline completely
- Gradually move the lens towards the eye while holding the upper and lower lid
- Give a final push to avoid dropping of lens
- To remove the lens, hold the upper edge of the lens with the upper lid and remove the suction by pressing the lower edge with the lid. The other method is to use a plunger. Attach the plunger in the inferior part of the lens at 6 o'clock position using suction and pull the lens outwards.

Complications that can be faced in scleral lens fitting are: Air bubbles (center or periphery), bulbar redness, conjunctival blanching and staining, conjunctival loose tissue, corneal staining, discomfort, giant papillary conjunctivitis, hypoxia and edema, lens adhesion, microbial keratitis and infiltrate, mucus and debris, neovascularization and vision problems.

Rose K Lenses

These are modified RGP lenses which are designed for irregular corneas like various grades of keratoconus, pellucid marginal degeneration, Terrien marginal degeneration and post-surgical corneal abnormalities. These lenses were named after an ophthalmologist Dr Paul Rose, who invented them. Rose K lenses provide better and comfortable vision correction in irregular corneas. Rose K lenses have the following properties which make it superior to the regular RGP lenses:

- Toric peripheral curves
- Asymmetric corneal technology: Helps in cases of 3 and 9 o'clock staining
- Front, back and bitoric designs
- Quadrant specific edge lifts—edge lift options are available other than standard edge which can also be quadrant specific.

Rose K lenses offer improved visual acuity, better comfort compared to other types of contact lenses, and the ability to delay or avoid the need for surgical intervention such as penetrating keratoplasty. Each individual gets a lens tailored to his corneal parameters. It ensures optimal fit, comfort and good visual acuity. However, they may not be suitable for some individuals . Some may find it challenging to adapt to wearing RGP lenses and in others, PK or scleral lenses may be a better option.

COMPLICATIONS OF CONTACT LENS

- **Hypoxic complications:** With soft contact lens there is only 1–2% of tear exchange with each blink. It is 10–20% with rigid gas permeable (RGP) or semisoft contact lens. This is known as adequate tear exchange. If contact lens is steep fitted or the D_K value is very low, or lens is very thick, oxygen supply to cornea is hampered and cornea starts becoming edematous with decreased sensations, superficial and deep vascularization, microcysts formation and superficial punctuate keratitis. Patient complains of redness in eyes, watering, blurring of vision and pain in eyes. Most common causes of hypoxia encountered clinically are overwear, steep fitted lens or patient sleeps with contact lens in eyes. So, patient must be advised not to sleep with contact lens in eyes.

Treatment: Remove the contact lens immediately and try to find out the cause, e.g.:

- Steep fitting, incomplete or inadequate blinking, patient slept with contact lens on, thick lens and poor quality material of contact lens with low DK value.
- Remove the cause and prescribe lubricating eye drops and topical antibiotics and call the patient after 3–4 days.

- **Infective complications:** Cornea may become infected with contaminated solution, lack of personal hygiene, use of tap water for contact lens storage or cleaning or from adjoining structures of eye. *Staphylococcus aureus, Acanthamoeba, Pseudomonas* are the common microorganisms which infect cornea. Patient complains of redness, watering, blurring of vision, pain in eyes. On slit lamp examination conjunctival congestion with purulent discharge may be seen. Cornea may show some infected lesion. Lack of compliance to instructions and delayed reporting predispose the patient to develop vision threatening complications.
  Treatment: Ask the patient to discontinue use of contact lens till further instructions. Take conjunctival swab and send for culture and sensitivity. Take history of using tap water for contact lens cleaning. Start antibiotics and lubricating eye drops and change the treatment if required as per culture report.
- **Allergic complications:** Patient may develop allergy to preservatives of contact lens solution. Very rarely he becomes allergic to contact lens material. He starts complaining of itching, redness, watering, etc. He may develop giant papillary conjunctivitis, follicular hypertrophy and hyperemia of conjunctiva.
  Treatment: Ask the patient to discontinue using contact lens for some time. Prescribe topical antihistaminics and diluted steroids. Once the symptoms are settled ask the patient to change the contact lens solution or the material as the case may be. He can also change the wearing schedule or lens design. He should be advised to use lubricating eye drops and clean his lenses regularly.
- **Giant papillary conjunctivitis:** It is papillary hyperplasia in the upper tarsal conjunctiva and occurs in 10–15% cases of soft contact lens users and 1–3% users of semisoft contact lens. Patient becomes aware of lens, complains of burning sensation, blurred vision, intolerance to contact lens, mucinous discharge and drooping of upper eyelid.

Treatment: Stop using contact lens for at least a few months. Use lubricating eye drops and diluted steroids, sodium cromoglycate eye drops and vasoconstrictor eye drops.

- **Traumatic complications:** Patient may sustain injury with contact lens edge or finger nail while inserting or removing the contact lens. This may cause redness of eyes, watering and FB sensation of eyes.
  Treatment: Fluorescein staining should be done and area of injury should be drawn on prescription slip for future reference. Stop using contact lens for some time. Remove any eyelash or foreign body from eye if any. Prescribe antibiotics and lubricating eye drops for 4–5 days.
- **Deposits:** They are most common with soft contact lens, more with extended wear than daily wear and least common with hard contact lens. Deposits consist of calcium and proteins from tears and cleaning solutions. Deposits impair oxygen permeability, interfere with vision. Lens surface becomes irregular and invites infection.
  Treatment: Patient should be advised to clean and disinfect contact lens regularly. Deposit prone patients should be advised to use semisoft lenses instead of soft contact lens and daily wear contact lens instead of extended wear contact lens.
- **Desiccation of cornea:** This is due to tear film disturbance caused by contact lens. Cornea may show 3–9 o'clock and 6 o'clock staining or dimple staining. Patient complains of redness, irritation, photophobia and intolerance to contact lens. 3–9 o'clock staining is caused by thick lens and 6 o'clock staining is caused by incomplete blinking. Dimple staining is due to tight fitting of contact lens.
  Treatment: Use a large lens of less thickness or a soft contact lens. Stress the need of complete blinking. Fitting of contact lens should be reassessed.
- **Toxic complications:** Certain drugs and preservatives of contact lens solution like benzalkonium chloride, thiomersal, etc., get deposited on contact lens surface and manifest as toxicity of cornea and conjunctiva. Patient complains of irritation, photophobia, watering, pain, etc.
  Treatment: Stop using contact lens for sometime. Change contact lens solution, clean and disinfect contact lens and use lubricating eye drops.

CONTACT LENS SOLUTIONS

Both soft and semisoft contact lenses require proper solutions for wetting, soaking and cleaning. Soft contact lens cannot be kept dry and must be stored in soft contact lens solutions. A contact lens solution is constituted by three agents namely wetting agent, soaking agent and cleaning agent.

- **Wetting agent:** It converts hydrophobic surface of contact lens into hydrophilic one. It acts as a cushion between lids and contact lens and contact lens and cornea. It stabilizes CL on finger tip due to capillarity action. Wetting agent is formed by:
  - Cushioning agent like polyvinyl alcohol
  - Preservatives like benzalkonium chloride and chlorobutanol
  - Wetting agent like polyvinyl alcohol
- **Soaking agent:** It keeps the lens in a state of hydration, maintains its sterility and removes mucus from surface of lens. Soaking agent is mainly constituted by preservatives like benzalkonium chloride. It prevents growth of gram +ve and gram –ve bacteria.
- **Cleaning agent:** A lens may get contaminated by oil, cosmetics, dried mucus, foreign body, etc. These things make the lens unfit for wearing because they irritate the eyes, blur the vision and act as a nidus for bacterial growth. Thus such a lens needs cleaning by:
  - **Friction rubbing:** Put the lens on palm with a drop of wetting agent and rub with finger tip. It can scratch the lens.
  - **Spray cleaning:** It is done by a specially designed kit.
  - **Hydraulic cleaning:** It is done by pumping action of water on contact lens in a special container.
  - **Ultrasonic cleaning:** It is done by passing ultrasonic waves in a fluid containing contact lens.

INDEX

Page numbers followed by *f* refer to figure, *fc* refer to flowchart, and *t* refer to table.

A

B

C

D

E

F

G

H

I

M

N

R

S

T

U

V

W

X

Y

Z